Contents

About the Publisher		iv
Reaching your Goal		v
Contributors		vi
Abbreviations		ix
Foreword		x
Introduction		xii

Chapter 1	**The first year**	1
Chapter 2	**The second year**	43
Chapter 3	**The third year**	85
Chapter 4	**The fourth year**	127
Chapter 5	**The final year**	167
Chapter 6	**The intercalating year**	211

D0317976

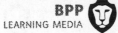

BPP
LEARNING MEDIA

About the Publisher

BPP Learning Media is dedicated to supporting aspiring professionals with top quality learning material. BPP Learning Media's commitment to success is shown by our record of quality, innovation and market leadership in paper-based and e-learning materials. BPP Learning Media's study materials are written by professionally-qualified specialists who know from personal experience the importance of top quality materials for success.

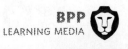

Reaching your Goal

The process of applying to medical school can be a somewhat long and arduous process but the rewards of a career within Medicine are infinite. BPP Learning Media and BPP University College School of Health are committed to supporting aspiring and current doctors to progress their career through our comprehensive range of books, personal development courses and degree programmes. I often say there is no other vocation that provides such breadth and depth of career options for the individual to follow and specialise in. Whether it is the fast paced nature of the A&E department or the measured environment of Pathology, there is something for everyone.

There is no greater privilege than being responsible for leading the treatment of patients and sharing in their recovery. There are few other careers that provide such diversity on a daily basis. A passion for helping others, clear communication skills especially empathy, excellent team working and leadership qualities as well as the ability to strike a work-life balance are all skills that an accomplished doctor should possess.

The decision to follow a career in Medicine is something that should not be taken lightly and you should undertake careful research to ensure it really is for you. A career in Medicine is not for everyone and I would urge readers to ensure they have undertaken sufficient work experience to gain a balanced insight into what becoming a doctor really entails.

I first began mentoring aspiring medical students seven years ago when it was clear that many individuals were not gaining access to the help and support they required to successfully apply to medical school. It was with this in mind that I embarked on publishing our *Entry to Medical School Series* to provide a clear insight into the various facets of successfully getting into medical school. Whether it is help with choosing the right medical school, how to prepare an outstanding personal statement or how to succeed in your medical school interview, our comprehensive range of books provide the advice that is so often hard to find.

I would like to take this opportunity to wish you the very best of luck with applying to medical school and hope that you pass on some of the gems of wisdom that you acquire along the way to other aspiring medics.

Matt Green
Series Editor – Entry to Medical School
Director of Professional Development – BPP University
College of Professional Studies

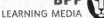

BPP 🦁
LEARNING MEDIA

v

Contributors

Chapter 1

Jade Woolley
Southampton University

Finn Morgan Taplin
Plymouth University

Teodora Filipescu
University of St Andrews

Nina Shavel
University of Cambridge

Ruth Collins
Swansea University

Chapter 2

Gareth Wilson
Kings College London

Sana ullah Khan
University of East Anglia

Michael Hale
University of Warwick

John Shenouda
University of Sussex

Michael William Mather
Durham University

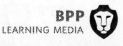

Chapter 3

Syed Muhammad Tahir Nasser
University College London

Emma Gees
University of Leeds

Penelope Cresswell
Cardiff University

LE Dawson
University of York

Leyla Swafe
University of Aberdeen

Chapter 4

Stephen Barratt
University of Sheffield

Neil Chanchlani
University of Birmingham

Thomas Kwan
Keele University

Kristina Lee
University of Edinburgh

Ross Kenny
University of Nottingham

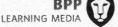

Chapter 5

Zuliana K Banda
Newcastle University

Dr Thomas Wood
Oxford University

Dr Ban Sharif
St George's, University of London

Dr Douglas H Blackwood
University of Glasgow

Dr Sheetal Patel
Barts and The London

Chapter 6

Lucy Robinson
Cardiff University

Shahana Hussain
Leicester University

Jonathan Chun-Hei Cheung
Imperial College London

Rathy Ramanathan
University of Liverpool

Fabienne Verrall
University of Bristol

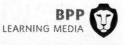

Abbreviations

A levels	Public examination in a secondary school subject, used as qualification for entrance into a university
ANP	Atrial Natriuretic Peptide
BMAT	BioMedical Admissions Test
BMJ	British Medical Journal
DGH	District General Hospital
EMQs	Extended Matching Questions
EWTD	European Working Time Directive
GAMSAT	Graduate Australian Medical School Admission Test
GCSE	General Certificates of Secondary Education
GMC	General Medical Council
GP	General Practitioner
HEMS	Helicopter Emergency Medical Service
KT	Knowledge Test
MB	Bachelor of Medicine
MBBS	Bachelor of Medicine, Bachelor of Surgery
MCQs	Multiple Choice Questions
MOSLER	Multi-station Objective Structured Clinical Examination Record
MSF	Médecins Sans Frontières
MTAS	Medical Training Application Service
NHS	National Health Service
OSCEs	Objective Structured Clinical Examinations
OSLER	Objective Structured Long Examination Record
OSPE	Objective Structured Practical Examinations
PBL	Problem Based Learning
PPD	Personal and Professional Development
SAQs	Short Answer Questions
SSS	Student Selected Study
UKCAT	UK Clinical Aptitude Test
USMLE	United States Medical Licensing Examination

Foreword

So do you want to be a brain surgeon? Do you want to explore the intricate synaptic workings of the brain, to stimulate sensations; or do you want to heal hearts, reactivating the impulses in Purkinje fibres that ensure there still is, a pulse to keep your finger on. Or perhaps you would like to eradicate cancers, to irradiate or resect carcinomas. Whatever specialty you choose, you will: one day join a fraternity of fellow physicians, who have the unique privilege of being people worthy of being entrusted with the lives of all and sundry. Before embarking on this journey it is vital to take measure of oneself: before being measured by panels of others, for the journey ahead is that of a lifetime, for even Professors remain students of Medicine!

This highly valuable book is a portal into the first part of that journey a period during which you will submit yourself to be lead along paths, to learn the basis of the terrain, the shapes of the fields, valleys and hills. You will learn how to read the maps of the medical world.

The journey ahead is arduous for most. You will need the stamina, perseverance, patience and passion to mount the pinnacle of qualification as a doctor. The path ahead certainly has many obstacles in the form of exams and assessments and perhaps even ravines that will catch out the unwary. Despite this, to forever keep your eye on the path alone will detract from the beauty of the terrain all around you and the passage of the moments of your life with your new companions. Few doubt that life at Medical School and University encompass some of the best days of your life.

This is a unique book, the first of its kind that collates the first hand experiences of real travellers at different stages of the journey through medical school. You will find that they do come in all shapes, sizes, ages and backgrounds: some are experienced climbers while others are perhaps just learning to walk unaided! Their 'warts n all' rough guide will help you make the biggest decision any traveller has to make: whether or not this is the right journey for you: something that only you can decide! The authors of this book are to be congratulated for sharing their insights and enabling the reader to grasp the realities of medical school life in terms of the many and varied curricula as well as extra-curricular life.

BPP
LEARNING MEDIA

Many of the authors have now qualified and have experienced the sensation of momentary elation on the peak of the mountain they seemed to forever climb, a peak from which they can now survey the vast expanse of the 'real' medical world within which they will carve their careers!

M Asif Chaudry

MA BM BCh Oxon MD MRCS(Eng) FRCS(Gen.Surg)

Oesophagogastric Surgeon
St Thomas' Hospital

Surgical Research Fellow
University College London

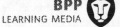

Introduction

Are *you* interested in medicine? Would you like to know what medical school is all about? If so, then you've picked up the right book... a first of its kind!

It's hard for me to believe that this endeavour has finally come to fruition. When I first got the idea for this book as a final year medical student, I wanted to tell the stories of medical students in the hope of stripping away any illusions and revealing the truth about medical training. I was not interested in giving you advice to enhance your chances for admission to medical school, instead I wanted to uncover what lies in store for you once you get in! Medical schools in the UK are notoriously difficult to get into, and it seems only to be getting harder. Nonetheless, many dream of pursuing a career in medicine, not knowing if it is best suited for them or what lies ahead. It only makes sense to spend some time thinking about what you should expect and what you really want from a medical school.

What is life really like as a medical student? That is the question! I endeavour to answer this all-important question in what I feel is the best possible way: by looking into the lives of medical students at different levels of training from across the UK. The 30 contributors are from different walks of life and include international and intercalating students, mature and graduate students, access course students, as well as public and private school entrants. Consequently, the content of this book is 100% student-led. It is written by medical students for anyone interested in pursuing a career in medicine. After all, we are in the best and unique position to tell you what you need to know!

Each one of us shares our personal experiences, career aspirations and reflections. We tell our story in our own words offering invaluable insight and a close-up look at medical training. The different tales consist of candid reports and a variety of viewpoints and so I invite you to read on and you will be transported into our lives. We are eager to share with you the highs and lows of medical school. You also get the student perspective on the structure of the different medical courses from across the country. It is then up to you to decide on the 'takehome' messages.

Although I strongly believe that reading these personal stories is a great way to find out more about medical education, it is important that you get the perspective of other medical students as well as more senior

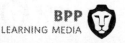

colleagues such as foundation programme trainees, registrars and consultants, whose experiences after medical school and on the job are also invaluable and so please bear these in mind when considering a career in medicine. I therefore strongly encourage you to not only read this book, but also to seek a range of different views in order to get a balanced account of what medical school is like.

Finally, the life of a medical student is known for being challenging but is also an immensely rewarding experience... I will not say any more on the topic! Instead, I will let the following stories speak for themselves. I promise you that these tales will change your assumptions about medical education and will hopefully help you make better-informed decisions regarding your career aspirations.

I wish you the best of luck with everything.

Dr Sihame Benmira

FY2
Guy's and St Thomas' NHS Foundation Trust

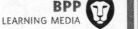

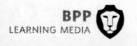

Chapter 1

The first year: A dose of reality from five medical students

Jade Woolley

Nina Shavol

Finn Morgan Taplin

Ruth Collins

Teodora Filipescu

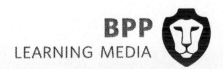

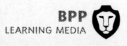

The first year: A dose of reality from five medical students

'There's no 'typical' medical student, and applicants shouldn't be discouraged by not having the standard formula of education, vocational epiphany, work experience and convenient extra-curricular skills'

Name: Jade Woolley
Age: 19
University: Southampton University
Course: Medicine and BMedSc (BM5) (5 years)
Year: 1
Extra info: I lived most of my life outside the UK in army camps

I started medical school in 2010, having just finished my A levels at school (I thought if I had a five-year degree coming up I'd best make a start as soon as possible!). My father is in the British Forces, so I've spent most of my life living outside the UK in army camps. I did my GSCEs and A levels in a Service Children's Education school in Germany, and spent some time living in the United States before that. Coming to university was the first time I'd lived in England for eleven years, so it was quite a big change! Quite simply, I'd like to share my experiences of my first year at medical school in the hope that it might be useful to others thinking of applying.

How it all started

I first considered a career in medicine during the lower sixth: it wasn't something I'd wanted to do since time immemorial (so there was no danger putting that cliché in my personal statement!). I fancied a job that would allow me to be at the forefront of something scientific and exciting; I was captivated by the books of Robert Winston and Oliver Sacks, and the versatility of medicine struck me as a brilliant springboard for anything I wanted to do in the future. This was probably a bit idealistic, but pursuing a vocational, practical career was certainly important for me.

For a long time I tried to dissuade myself from applying – I didn't fancy the hassle, the extra tests were complicated to arrange, being stuck with no offers would scupper me for a year and a hundred other excuses ran through my head. Annoyingly though, I knew I'd be kicking myself for eternity if I didn't at least try, and I felt particularly sure I'd never be really satisfied doing anything else.

It's fair to say I was, and probably still am, a little bit vague about why exactly I want to do medicine, and one can feel that that's a huge disadvantage in applying. I dreaded the interview question 'why do you want to become a doctor?' because it seemed impossible to explain my fairly esoteric incentives, but I increasingly feel that this is quite justifiable and people shouldn't be deterred by not knowing their exact motivation.

Application

I once heard the UCAS application described as the 'most soul-destroying time of your life.' Unfortunately, I would completely agree.

I was the only one in my school applying to medicine and the first for quite a few years, which made finding people to ask for advice a tad more tricky. My school Exams Officer had never heard of the BMAT, I had to travel to Brussels to take the UKCAT and there were no resources or guidebooks available for me to beg and borrow. I couldn't afford to travel to the UK to take entrance exam revision courses and am glad I didn't – I'm sceptical of the value of any of these tests, and really do feel that they're just another layer of box-ticking at vast expense to the candidate.

Sorting out work experience was incredibly difficult on an army camp – take the usual hospital reticence in accepting students, then add some layers of military secrecy and confidentiality. In the end I was incredibly lucky and a friend helped me arrange three weeks' observation in operating theatres at a local German hospital. This was a fantastic experience, if captured by me only through my limited snippets of German and nurse's kind translations. It proved that medical schools aren't lying in saying it's not what you do, it's what you get from it!

Eventually I managed to meld together an application, which was solidly rejected from three of the places I applied to (Bristol, Oxford and Peninsula). Waiting with no offers, no idea what you're going to do if you get another rejection and the prospect of all your future plans disappearing is a horrible thing to do, especially during your A levels. I wouldn't wish it on anybody, and it was with enormous relief that I finally received an offer from Southampton!

Life as a first year medical student

My typical day as a first year started with a 9.00am lecture (this became increasingly hard to get up for as the year went on). Our lectures were split between the university campus and the General Hospital, which meant lots of cycling every morning – the soundest advice I can give to Southampton medics is to get a bicycle! Generally, each day had about four- or five-hour-long lectures, with just enough time to dash for a cup of tea in between.

BPP
LEARNING MEDIA

Our timetable varied massively every week but, in addition to lectures, the year group would be divided into thirds for sessions in the histology and anatomy labs once or twice a week. There were pathology, physiology and pharmacology smaller group tutorials built into the course, which were excellent for consolidating topics from lectures. Course tutorials, focused on the body system we were studying, were a brilliant opportunity to get help and ask questions, usually completely off topic!

We had fortnightly visits to local GP practices, where we could speak to patients and put into practice some of what we were learning in lectures. I found these brilliant – a few hours at the GPs seeing patients, discussing conditions and messing about with stethoscopes (and, of course, making tea) would buoy me up for the subsequent two weeks of dry lectures.

Our compulsory workload was fairly small: each semester we were set a major essay to complete, and there were shorter reflective accounts for our student selected and inter-professional learning units. The bulk of the work was in preparation for tutorials and anatomy sessions, which you needed to do to get the most out of them. Overall, I think the workload was manageable – I would do roughly two hours on weekday evenings and five on weekends, but this was very flexible. It's most important to just ensure you don't get too behind.

The main assessment for the first year was in the form of big scary end-of-semester exams. There were three papers for each semester (multiple-choice, long answer and an anatomy practical). I quite liked the method of assessment – we were offered opportunities to give feedback to external examiners, and it felt fair. Our final grade considered our exams, student-selected units, basic history-taking and essay performances.

Social life

There's truth in the cliché that medics work hard and play hard. Although I'm not a big party-goer, I know there are plenty of opportunities for those who are, and you definitely don't sacrifice social life in studying medicine. Nevertheless, striking a balance and carefully choosing what you do is key. I got involved in Southampton's medical society (MedSoc), who put on excellent socials to fit our hectic schedules and organised some brilliant charity events.

Getting involved with societies run by medical students was the perfect way I could enjoy a social life that didn't detract from work, and was handy for getting a few hints from the older years! There were loads of things to do that were superb fun and really valuable: I loved being part of Teddy Bear Hospital, teaching young children not to be afraid of doctors, and it looks excellent on your CV (or

MTAS). The only problem I had was not having enough time to devote to all the fantastic initiatives that medical students can join!

Expectations versus reality

It's hard to say whether the reality of medical school met my expectations, having had no prior experience of medicine or university. I expected to have learnt more clinical things in my first year, but I understand the need for some solid academic background first! I was surprised by the format of teaching – I'd not realised I'd be spending all day every day sat in lectures for hours on end. Nevertheless, there were things that exceeded my expectations, such as the variety of activities you can engage in and the opportunity to see some patients. There's also the really supportive atmosphere amongst medical students, which I hadn't anticipated but am very grateful for!

What I love about medical school

Being a medical student. This is a bit egotistical, but it is fantastic! You can take enormous pride in your crammed timetable, ironed shirts and shiny 'Medical Student' badge. The general public still have an immense respect for doctors, and it's a huge privilege to be on the receiving end of some of that.

Diversity. I was pleasantly surprised the immense variety of backgrounds that people on my course had. It felt like only a handful was straight from school; many had taken gap years or were mature students with a real wealth of experience. I could start the morning with somebody who'd decided to do medicine after finishing her nursing degree, then sit next to a Microbiology graduate (vital for some of our infection lectures!), chat with the Economics graduate and then attend a tutorial with an ex-policewoman. Being amongst such an assortment was fascinating.

Atmosphere. Before starting medical school I'd heard a lot about medics being horribly competitive. Luckily, in my experience, this is completely untrue! There was a wonderfully relaxed atmosphere in my year – I think everybody was so glad to be there that they didn't care how well they were doing compared to anybody else. Nobody pestered you for your exam grades or boasted about theirs, and it was an agreeable contrast to what I'd expected. While academic performance is obviously important, I've come to realise being a 'well-rounded' individual with lots of pursuits and interests is just as valuable in making you a good medical student. There were excellent support networks too, including the senior pastoral tutor, your personal tutor, the MedSoc welfare rep, and of course your friends! Everybody was conscious of looking out for each other, and it was comforting to know you were in a really supportive environment.

Patients. Early patient contact wasn't something I'd specifically looked for when applying, but I now think it's essential. Just seeing a tiny

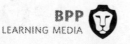

fraction of proper medicine was a real incentive to help me through lectures, and some of the patients met were incredibly helpful. Getting a snapshot of somebody's life, job, past and their future feels like a real honour, and reminds you that there's more to medicine than just science.

Subjects. The subjects that you're exposed to in your pre-clinical years are daunting in their volume and breadth (especially looking at your recommended reading list!), but I loved getting a little glimpse into each area. A series of lectures would cover anatomy, histology, pharmacology, biochemistry, microbiology and pathology, taking all the bits that were relevant to the system we were studying. There aren't many degrees where one minute you hold aloft a heart in anatomy, and the next take beta-blockers and measure your blood pressure in a pharmacology practical!

What I hate about medical school

Size. Admittedly, mine isn't a large medical school, but going from A level classes of four or five to lecture halls of nearly 200 is a big shock. You can't really pop your hand up mid-lecture and ask for something to be repeated, like you might have done at school! It was disconcerting to devote lots of time and energy towards material delivered by a lecturer who doesn't even know you exist, and certainly won't know your name. This wasn't always the case though – tutors and lecturers in small group sessions got to know you a bit better, and getting stuck into lectures by answering questions or volunteering for things helped too. I tried to do this whenever possible, and so far I've been electrocuted (something to do with action potentials), had my eye movements tracked while describing my toothbrush (communication skills), thrown rugby balls into bin bags (in manner of liver enzymes) and been wrapped in a bed sheet (to demonstrate the peritoneum, obviously). Aside from being great fun, this does help things stick in your memory and I'd highly advocate active participation!

Death by PowerPoint. As I say, being proactive can alleviate the drudgery of this somewhat, but it's still a drag. And unbelievably soporific.

Timetable. Compared to the world of work and my (hopefully) future job, the 9.00 to 4.00-ish days of my first year were fairly indolent. It didn't seem like this, though, when the rest of the university and my non-medic friends had so few lectures they had whole days off midweek and 9.00am starts were unheard of. It was easy to become distanced from the university proper because of timetable and the medic 'bubble', but personally I quite enjoyed the sense of self-sufficiency.

Exams. Obviously, exams are an unavoidable part of your training. This doesn't mean you can't detest them though! Spending every holiday in ardent revision is nobody's idea of a good time, especially when you're just rote-memorising huge amounts of facts. I suppose it pays off in the end.

Most valuable experience

My most valuable experiences so far have been ones involving seeing patients. It's difficult to pin down a specific instance, as I think you appreciate something different every time you meet someone, try out your history taking skills and listen to them.

Nevertheless, a recent experience with a hospitalised, 67-year-old patient admitted with lumbar pain stands out particularly for me. It was the first time my colleagues and I had tried taking a history in a ward, and we spent half an hour quizzing him inexpertly about what pain he'd had, what drugs he'd taken, whether he was employed and all the standard questions. He was a nice old chap, declared he'd never had any illness in his life and then wished us well with our studies. Later on I asked the doctor what was wrong with him and she told me he had advanced renal cancer, with only about six months to live. Suddenly realising this made me think completely differently about him – it was poignantly sad that he was nearing the end of his life so abruptly, but it was also remarkable that he'd spoken to me perfectly calmly as I'd fumbled through my history questions, so courageously having come to terms with his illness. This was undoubtedly something I'll never forget, and it was a tremendous privilege to experience.

Least valuable experience

My least valuable experience of medical school was right at the beginning, during our anatomy sessions. We were given a huge booklet of bones, muscles, nerves and blood supplies to memorise, and I wandered around the cadavers not having a clue what to look for or what anything meant. It was extremely demoralising to feel completely overwhelmed by all that we needed to know, especially when the specimens were so crowded round you couldn't see anything anyway and it was difficult to get help. Luckily, this got a lot better as time went on – I found an excellent pair of friends to quiz me, and we could take our time and go back to the lab outside of timetabled sessions when everything was quieter. Nevertheless, that feeling of rather helpless despondency can be quite easy to slip into, and it's vital to make sure you don't!

The future

I'd hope I'm quite relaxed about the future. I've no burning ambition to enter a particular field, and certainly haven't enough experience to make an informed judgement. There are a few things I think I'll eliminate: my total conceptual inability to grasp embryology makes me feel that perhaps that's not my future vocation! I do idly entertain a vision of me as a country GP in some remote rural corner in the future (at least according

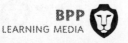

to my housemates), and I reckon I'd be happy if that's what I was doing in ten years' time. Working abroad is something that I'm really keen on doing, especially within Europe. It's a great advantage to medicine that there are so many career pathways and options available to give you lots of scope for the future, and I want to try to make the most of them.

I hope, reading this, hesitant prospective medics would be encouraged to apply. There's no 'typical' medical student, and applicants shouldn't be discouraged by not having the standard formula of education, vocational epiphany, work experience and convenient extra-curricular skills (though there's nothing wrong with this!). I think it's also perfectly normal to not be quite sure exactly why you want to do medicine, and my experiences as a first-year student have shown me that it really grows on you with time.

Ten things I wish I had known before starting medical school

1. There's a lot of rote memorisation to do. Although it's essential, it can be quite difficult to do when you don't feel like you have enough background knowledge in the subject to start with.

2. There will be early starts. All the time. And late finishes.

3. You'll be working a lot harder than your friends doing other degrees.

4. Most of your teaching will be done in a lecture theatre.

5. It's a long time until you're able to do anything exciting.

6. You will meet medical students who will be your friends for life, and medical students who you can't believe are going to be future doctors!

7. You'll get medical student hypochondria, where you think you'll be bizarrely inflicted with every disease you're studying.

8. It's fine to constantly question your motivation in wanting to be a doctor.

9. It's easy to become bogged down in lectures; remember they don't last for ever.

10. It's important to not work too hard, and make sure you spend time doing the things you enjoy!

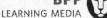

Practical Guidance Tips

- The endless lectures in the first few years can really wear you out – nobody wants to be sat in silence in a dark lecture theatre for five hours of their day, practically every weekday. Try to keep motivated by getting involved as much as you can, answering questions and sitting near the front (yes, I think it really does help!).

- Get involved with your medical society! They put on fabulous events, provide welfare, help you get to know people from all walks of life and do loads for charity: if in doubt, ask MedSoc!

BPP
LEARNING MEDIA

'Due to my seemingly innate inability to back away from a challenge, I found my circumstances not to be an insurmountable obstacle, but perhaps the perfect motivating tool.'

Name: Finn Morgan Taplin
Age: 20
University: Plymouth University
Course: Five-year Bachelor of Medicine, Bachelor of Surgery (BM, BS)
Year: 1
Extra info: Took a gap year, rather unusually, at the age of 16

To put it quite bluntly, despite the deceptively liberal attitude of our modern age, it remains incredible to me how difficult it is to traverse beyond the level of society to which we were seemingly assigned at birth. I was raised on a narrowboat, and from a relatively early age I was aware of the way that many viewed our lifestyle. With our lack of electricity, running water and modern appendages, opinions ranged from 'quaint and romantic' to 'backwards' and I remember quite vividly the way in which expectations of me, from school and from my peers, were adjusted accordingly. I have chosen to contribute to this book because I feel passionately that our background should never be allowed to define us. I feel that the choices of our parents, however well they may have been intended, are still heavily conjoined to our prospects. If I can achieve one thing by sharing my experiences, I would like to motivate somebody to open their eyes and see no plateau to their opportunities. Life is what you make of it, so depend only on yourself and invent your own luck.

How it all started

I have, and have always had, a seemingly infinite thirst for knowledge – particularly knowledge in its rawest form. We are after all an agglutination of cells (albeit acutely arranged) and chemical components with an electric spark of sentience. This idea has consistently amazed me to such a degree that it has often been at the heart of my questioning.

My motivation for choosing medicine specifically is a more complex issue, as I fell rather head over heels for Mathematics until well into my GCSE years. I was quite taken by the purity of it, and its mechanical, almost beautiful mixture of complexity and logical simplicity. I never realistically considered a career in mathematics however, due to the fact that I felt it was always lacking a little in the human aspect, that would have given it passion and dynamic, real application. If I had to assign

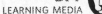

mathematics a colour, I fear that it would be grey – perfectly pleasant, but essentially cold and emotionally stunted. Medicine on the other hand, I feel would be a loud, gaudy scarlet: emotive, human, but at the same time bursting with the most fiendishly complex aspects of science and technology. I chose medicine almost entirely for the academic interest in people rather than for the more obvious, healthcare aspects. Engrained in my mind since the dawn of my understanding has been the image of a doctor as a scientist, a psychologist, and a teacher – but this idea alone I found to be a little lacking in substance. People are so incredibly complex – difficult and stubborn beyond physical measure, but laced with compassion and empathy. A potent infusion of science, and these human qualities felt too intriguing to let go.

Application

When applying to read medicine, you discover the truly frightening meaning of 'all or nothing'. There is no escaping that the whole process (with an honourable mention of the UKCAT at this point) is detrimental to sanity. To narrow down all of your potential paths of life into five discrete choices is something that I would not wish on any sentient being.

It is a strange feeling to be so in control, and so lost. Sitting in the library of my college two days before the application deadline, having researched every conceivable aspect of every UK medical institution, I have to say that the method that I employed to choose my universities was only tenuously linked to rationality. I chose Nottingham because I knew that they employed dissection as a tool for learning anatomy, and I was morbidly fascinated by this idea; Peninsula because I fell in love with the idea of the small group teaching and emphasis on independent learning, and Bristol because, truthfully, they did not involve the UKCAT in the application process.

I was interviewed at Nottingham and at the Plymouth campus of Peninsula. In preparing for these it has to be said that my borderline obsessive tendencies came into their own. I devoured every conceivable piece of literature on medical school interviews, and begged my GP for all of her back issues of the BMJ. Having covered up all of my exposed tattoos with appropriately placed neck-ties and bracelets, I made the resolution to speak candidly and with an honest vehement.

I received conditional offers from both of the interviews I attended, but my final choice of institution was actually based upon the two vastly different interviews that I experienced: at Nottingham, I was seated on one side of an expansive oak desk. In front of the two gentlemen that sat across from me, was a copy of my personal statement, annotated in red by an unfamiliar hand. While one asked me about my opinions regarding the ethical issues surrounding euthanasia, the other gazed skywards with a

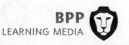

kind of passionate apathy. The first spoke as though his words were bullets, his mouth an automatic weapon. I felt every silence as my tone trailed off, uncertain due to the absence of any facial expressions on their behalf.

At Peninsula, I was given a cup of tea and invited to join a collection of doctors, university professors and a member of the public for an 'academic chat'. I was so struck by the way in which that they regarded my opinions as those of a peer that I was able to open up beyond my nervousness and speak with vigor and intelligence. I feel that I did not have to tick any boxes so to speak, and even though this was most likely not the case, the freedom that I felt manifested itself in a lively and intellectual debate.

Life as a first year medical student

On meeting my peers for the first time, I was struck by the fact that everybody was very sure of their own identity. Striving so hard and for so long to stand out and be noticed among the herd of faceless applicants forces you to develop a very strong sense of self, and a razor sharp awareness of your own opinions as well as your limitations.

A typical day is defined by how early the lectures start. After pushing aside the fuzzy head from the night before, the likelihood of breakfast is defined by weighing up the benefits of a full stomach versus snatching a few more precious minutes in bed. We follow a two-week timetable, and although at first glance this appears to be fairly modest in terms of hours, the emphasis is very much on self-directed learning, of which we are expected to do between 15 and 20 hours per week. Our terms are organised so that we follow a series of case units, each lasting for two weeks. These are realistic clinical scenarios that encompass elements of anatomy, physiology, biochemistry and pharmacology, which we identify and discuss during our group 'problem-based learning' (PBL) sessions and research in our own time. In terms of quantifying our schedule, in a two-week period we have ten hours of lectures related to our case unit, four hours of PBL, four hours of 'Clinical skills' (in which we learn skills such as venepuncture, physical examinations and injection techniques), and six hours of 'Life Sciences' in which we are taught anatomy and physiology in an intense, didactic fashion. Once every fortnight we have a two-hour community placement, allowing us to experience healthcare both in a traditional sense such as a GP surgery, and alternative treatments such as acupuncture or music therapy.

Social life

The stereotypical medical student works hard and plays harder. I can categorically say that this is true. As soon as the timetable has been analysed, appropriate late nights can be planned to cause the least collateral damage in terms of early lectures. In the first few terms at least, sleep is overrated. There is no escaping the fact that studying Medicine carries with it a certain intensity, and if not carefully diffused, the stress levels can become unbearable.

I joined the university lacrosse team early on, in part for fitness, but also to escape from other medical students. At any social gathering that we have as a faculty, the conversations tend towards medicine at an alarming rate. I am keen to avoid this at all costs, as it is impossible to remain motivated academically, if our social time involves as much medicine as our weekdays. I believe that this tendency is responsible for the very real risk of burnout that can manifest in the case of an imbalance. I am of the opinion that there are some elements of our lives that must remain isolated from medicine, lest we risk our own sanity. In addition, we all have bad days. Believe me, there is no frustration that you can't sweat out.

Expectations versus reality

My expectations of medical school were formulated almost entirely in my own mind, having known nobody personally that had gone through the process before. I found A levels hard, and my thinking was that if they were the stepping stone to get here in the first place, medicine itself would be borderline impossible. While there is no doubt that medicine is challenging, it is so in a rather inoffensive way, more a stretching of the mind than a mental annihilation. In reality, you are supported and taught to change your learning approach in order to deal with the more difficult concepts, and while at A level each subject forms a separate entity, medicine is a single broad subject within which the subsections are all linked. The other expectation that I had was that all medical students would be for the most part straight laced perfectionists. I am however delighted to inform you that never in my life have I met such an intriguingly deviant group of people. Everybody has a spark of oddness and such a wonderful depth, perhaps it is the awareness of identity that I mentioned earlier, but whatever the reason it makes for an electric dynamic in group sessions and within each year group as a whole.

What I love about medical school

As with many of my fellows, my competitive attitude is innate. I thrive under pressure, and the more I am told that I cannot do something, the more I crave to prove myself. For this reason, I love the fact that nothing in medicine is stoic – you have to throw your whole self into it or quickly be left in the dust. Far from creating rivalries, this charged atmosphere commands a sense of community; medical students stick together because we see a little of ourselves in each other, and I find this to be both comforting and motivating.

I have been honoured to share my time so far with a group of friends that have become so close as to be indistinguishable from family. I believe that the intense environment in which we exist has the remarkable ability to either destroy friendships or irreversibly cement them.

What I hate about medical school

As with the students that colonise it, there is nothing about medical school that can be considered average. Things are either 'wonderful', 'terrible', or a lively cocktail of the two. Among some students (but by no means all or even a majority) the sheer ego is palpable. At risk of making a stark generalisation, I would have to say that it is the male medics who steal the crown for those most likely to develop a debilitating God complex!

The competitive element, which is positive in so many ways, can honestly become unpleasant when taken to the extreme. When exam time comes, the emphasis is so much on individual success that all sense of peer support goes out of the window. The sense of community for the most part evaporates, and an individual's own notes and learning materials are coveted beyond belief. I think that this is because the mentality of seeing everybody else as a potential threat has been ingrained since the application process, but the death grip with which many of us still hold onto it will hopefully relax with time.

Most valuable experience

While on a clinical placement, I witnessed a consultation in which a lady presented with a history of failure to conceive. She was profoundly overweight, and entered the room with fierce presence. Having been told that her trouble was due predominantly to her weight, she denied in outraged tones any possible connection between the two. By her own admission, she considered herself 'damaged goods' having tried every diet and exercise programme suggested by healthcare professionals, all of which had failed her.

The way in which the doctor reached her was by making the white hot issue of her weight secondary. If she was to conceive a healthy child, she would have to be healthy herself inside and out. Motivating her to change her behaviour through care of her potential child gave her the autonomy to act, rather than to be told.

I came to the conclusion that how she spoke was a polar opposite to how she perceived herself. A coping mechanism for such self loathing is perhaps to project blame and hurt onto any third party, to give oneself a few seconds of tenuous relief. The reasons behind her damaged psyche remained a mystery to me in the slender ten minutes of the consultation, but I realise that if we judge only what we see, we inevitably neglect the problem at its root. By observing such stark self hatred, it became clear that the physical symptoms were secondary.

Least valuable experience

Self diagnosis is an interesting phenomenon that while not unique to medical students is most certainly prevalent among them; a product perhaps of being surrounded by a foray of rare and exciting illnesses, many with non-specific profiles. I spent an uncomfortable three days reading about respiratory tract infections in preparation for our first serious exam, and was worked up into an asthmatic fervor by the well meaning concern of friends, when I developed a mild cough and a psychosomatic shortness of breath. Having crashed back to reality fairly swiftly, I am of the opinion that our sanity is dependent on a level of disconnect.

The future

Since first considering medicine as a career, I have felt that my future lies in surgery. I would like to work with my hands as well as my brain, and would relish the opportunity to hold a problem physically, and to solve it manually. Within this field, I am particularly drawn to facial reconstructive surgery. People lose their entire identity as a result of intent or accident, and giving such people back the ability to express themselves I believe is a valuable gift. Such fine movements of the knife re-sculpting emotive flesh, this delicacy belies the mechanistic, almost primal nature of surgery.

In ten years' time, whether I have changed my mind a thousand times as to my favoured route, I want to be challenged and tested as much as I feel I am today. As long as I can practise humane science with passion and flair, I will be content. I would never wish to remove myself from the human element of medicine, and so I am confident that my role will always be clinical.

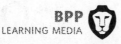

Ten things I wish I had known before starting medical school

1. Everybody genuinely is as frightened as you are; it is just a matter of how thick the veneer covering their insecurity happens to be.

2. The application process is tough, but it is tough for a reason. Universities need to be sure that successful students won't lose passion or burn out after a year or so. Passion cannot be taught, but medicine can.

3. The friends that you make at medical school will know you better than anybody ever has.

4. Sleep is a luxury, make the most of it pre-September.

5. Cherish any iota of genuinely free time you get.

6. Help is always available, but often it requires taking a little initiative: being proactive shows drive and determination, and this can only work in your favour.

7. Relevant work experience does not have to be a matter of shadowing the UK's top cardiac surgeon. If like me, your family has no medical connections, good clinical exposure can be harder to come by. It is not about what you've done, but what you have gained from it. If you can show that through a steady part-time job in an off-licence you have gained enviable interpersonal skills, and have demonstrated reliability and integrity, this will beat a clinical placement from which nothing was reflected upon hands down.

8. Weekends will quickly become a frenzied catch-up operation from the week before.

9. Competitiveness is prolific, concentrate on your own successes.

10. Finally, and I believe most importantly, obstacles exist only within the mind. Strength of thought and self belief can overcome literally any barrier.

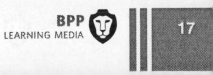

Practical Guidance Tips

- Commit: commit to your choices, and be stark and uncompromising with your ambitions. Aim high, and don't settle for less! As scary as it may seem, this is the one time where you have genuine autonomy, so use it.

- Throughout your application, do not be a faceless student with a bar code rather than an identity, be remembered. Voice an opinion, and justify it. Disagree. Debate. Don't be stereotypical, be unique.

BPP LEARNING MEDIA

> 'Everything can be achieved, provided the right amount of effort and passion is put in.'

Name:	Teodora Filipescu
Age:	20
University:	University of St Andrews
Course:	Six year programme – three pre-clinical years at University of St Andrews traditional programme plus three clinical years at another university
Year:	1
Extra info:	International European Union student

My name is Teodora and I am currently a first year medic at the University of St Andrews. Yet, my life had no connection with Scotland until quite recently. I was born in Romania, where I've lived and studied for the first 19 years of my life. In fact, my background is one of the reasons that determined me to share all my experiences in this book.

As a Romanian high school student, I found it extremely difficult to understand how to apply to a medical school in UK. PBL, UKCAT, BMAT and even A levels were all new concepts for me. I had no one to ask, no one to guide me and no one to offer me accurate information. I had to spend tens of hours in front of the computer trying to make sense of a completely new world, with different rules, traditions and values. Thus, obtaining a place in my first choice university came as a great surprise and relief to me. As a result, I decided to offer all my support to students in similar situations, for I know just how difficult and disheartening the application process can be. I hope that the following pages will give strength and courage to all those who are about to adventure towards such a challenging academic degree.

How it all started

My first thoughts regarding a medical career came at a very young age. Most people can imagine excited little girls consulting teddy bears with their plastic stethoscopes. Well, I suppose I was quite the opposite. Having two doctor grandparents around, it was not difficult for me to associate medicine with injections, regular consultations and blood tests. Medicine was neither fun nor exciting and I was determined to pursue any profession but the medical one.

Ironically, as I grew older, I discovered that biology was one of my favourite subjects and medicine didn't seem as frightening anymore. Of course, at that age all sciences are captivating enough to make one want

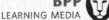

to become an architect, IT specialist, genetic researcher or even a novel writer! So there I was, weighing a handful of options, trying to decide what to do with my future.

Luckily, things became a lot clearer as I reached high school. Language classes were routine, maths was too complicated and my biology teacher was too lovely! It is amazing how a single person can change the course of one's life. A single amazing teacher influenced me in turning my interest into passion. I knew I wanted to participate in the Biology Olympiad after my first biology class and this desire was about to change my life.

Over the following four years I struggled to qualify to the national phase of the Olympiad. Failures only motivated me to work harder in order to achieve my goal. Older students became a model for me, my family and friends became supporters and my biology teacher – a mentor. By the time I finished high school, I understood that my results in the Olympiad competition were not the greatest achievement. What I actually gained from this experience was a real insight into the medical world – I understood anatomy, I did microscopic investigations, I took part in various teams and I was forced to perform under stressful conditions. Without realising it, my work helped me build up expectations for my future. At that point, I understood that I wanted to study medicine in a challenging environment. I wanted to compete with top students and, at the same time, to benefit from modern learning techniques and facilities. Thus, I decided to apply for a few UK medical schools that seemed to match my hopes.

Application

Choosing only four universities to apply to was a tough job. The greatest impediment was my Romanian qualification – the Romanian Baccalaureate – which, apparently, is not good enough for many UK medical schools. I was, thus, left with fewer options. I eventually applied to Oxford, Glasgow, Dundee and St Andrews. As I had a fifth choice left, I also applied to Edinburgh University for a genetic course, but I, like many other students, was actually determined to have a gap year, rather than start an unwanted degree. Even though all the universities I applied to had a good reputation and promoted themselves as being modern and up to date, St Andrews University caught my eye and heart from the very beginning.

After I submitted my application, the time passed painfully slowly. Proper sleep was only an abstract concept for me, and all I could do was calculate my chances for an interview. Sarcastically, no matter how much I tried to forget about my application, all the news, magazines and books seemed to remind me of my favourite university, especially given that the royal wedding was about to happen. Soon enough, I

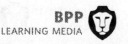

became a TSR (the student room) addict – checking the forums every few minutes, counting the people who had already received interviews and recalculating my chances once more. I could barely focus on my studies – which was probably the biggest mistake I made! – and the only comfort I had was the fact that I had not received a rejection.

Words cannot describe my happiness when I was offered three interviews in a two-week time interval. To top it up, the St Andrews interview came on the 23rd of December; what better Christmas gift could I have hoped for? Fortunately, I was conscientious enough to start preparation right away by reading specialised books and by doing mock interviews. Working hard is always the key to success, and interviews are no exception. Everything can be achieved, provided the right amount of effort and passion is put in.

Despite all the efforts to control my emotions, my first interview was a complete disaster. Indeed, Dundee's MMIs (multi-mini interviews) were not to my liking. I found it very difficult to completely forget one station and move forward to the next. There was no time to bond with the interviewers and the tasks were quite difficult for the amount of time we were given. While I do appreciate this method of interviewing, I think that some well prepared candidates cannot adapt to it. I am one of them.

My Glasgow and St Andrews interviews were very similar. Both were traditional, with a couple of interviewers chatting to me. I found it easier to develop a relationship with my dialog partners and I was able to expand my ideas; still, minding my answers as well as my posture and gestures was quite tricky! And, even though the interviews were almost the same, I managed to leave Glasgow smiling, while I could only cry after my St Andrews experience. I suppose it is never as bad as it seems – I got offers from both universities, making March of 2011 the happiest month of my life!

Overall, I think the application process was not only exciting, but fair as well. Interviewing applicants is a great opportunity to select the best students that would fit into that particular university environment. I think that applicants should always remember that if they get rejected, it is not because they are not valuable individuals, but because they do not fit into that environment. There is always a university out there that will exactly suit their personalities!

Life as a first year medical student

Medicine is tough even from the beginning of the training. Days can sometimes be monotonous – waking up at 8.00am, a rather decent hour, making my way to the university, spending between three and six hours in lectures, labs or clinical classes and coming back home only to find more work. There are eight lectures and six hours of seminars / tutorials / practicals each week; clinical case studies and clinical skills on a two-week cycle and up to six hours per week of directed self-learning ie guided studies. Even though the schedule might not seem too complicated, required reading can quickly pile up so I have to spend up to 30–35 hours a week reading and working on my guided studies. I find this manageable, as I enjoy most of the lectures and work is a way of satisfying my curiosity rather than a means to good exam results. At the end of the day, there are two to three hours of free time left for me to enjoy. I generally use this time to attend society meetings or other extra-curricular activities.

Of course, things can change dramatically during exams! I have to work my way through four exam periods a year – two mid semester assessments (MSA) and two end of semester assessments (ESA). Each exam period consists of four examinations. The grade that influences my degree is achieved by combining the results from a short written answers paper and a multiple choice paper. Besides these written papers, I also have to pass OSCE and OSPE exams, which test my clinical and practical abilities. From my point of view, the exams are very well structured as they are proportionate with the number of lectures and they always test every aspect of our module. The marking is precise and grading depends on the difficulty of the test, so that our result is actually representative for our knowledge. Overall, I am very pleased with the fairness of the exams, which is why I am always highly motivated to do my best in each paper.

Social life

Medical students have always complained that there is too much work, and too little time. While I agree with this statement, I do believe that time management can come in very handy. My personal strategy relies on doing most work during the week, while leaving a full free day during the weekend. I always have time to enjoy a good walk on the beach, a movie night or, occasionally, a nice party. Free time is relative to one's hobbies and entertainment methods, but as long as prioritisation takes place, combining hard work with fun is always possible!

Given the fact that I am generally a quiet person, moving away from home has actually made me more socially active. Not only do I go out more often, but I am also involved in three societies – the Surgical society, the Teddy Bear Hospital and Sexpression. Being part of such student groups is quite important to me. First of all, I was given the opportunity to attend talks or lectures offered by consultants from all over the UK. Second, but equally important, I got engaged in medical debates with my peers. As far as I am concerned, a balanced social life is formed of parties and concerts, as well as theatre plays and society meetings and I have managed to enjoy all of these in my first year as a medic.

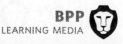

Expectations versus reality

Fortunately, the medical school I attend is everything I hoped for. The standard of teaching is high, the evaluation is accurate and my colleagues are quite an intellectual challenge. The University of St Andrews is rightly promoting its modern features! The new medical building is state of the art, with brand new lecture theatre, dissection room, clinical skills area and anatomy resource centre. The school is specially designed to offer access to information and the lecturers and demonstrators are always happy to chat to us, should we encounter any difficulties. In my case, reality overcame expectations.

What I love about medical school

There are many different aspects that I love about my medical school. To begin with, the spiral structure of the curriculum makes me feel that we accumulate information in an organised manner. On the initial turn of the spiral, fundamentally important knowledge is reviewed. During subsequent turns of the spiral, topics are revisited at a more advanced level and with increasing clinical application. The lectures are meant to offer a solid knowledge base, and due to the intercalated year included in our degree, we can fully understand the scientific base of Medicine. All of the academic staff is ready to support us not only intellectually, but morally as well. Asking questions is always praised and students are continuously encouraged to seek their own answers. In a word, the medical school's aim is to offer training rather than only degrees.

Most of the learning is done in a hands-on manner. Every lecture is reinforced through labs, practicals or dissection classes. Dissection in particular is extremely valuable. Seeing a real tissue or organ, being able to touch it and observe it is the easiest way to understand, rather than memorise anatomy. '*Thinking is more interesting than knowing, but less interesting than looking*' (Johann Wolfgang von Goethe).

Innovation is a word that perfectly characterises the learning experience. For example, the clinical skills area is equipped with tens of modern cameras; we are encouraged to film ourselves practising our skills, to review the videos and to learn from our own mistakes. The same technique is used for communication skills classes, when we practise our history taking abilities. Reflecting is clearly important, and the medical school does all that is possible to stimulate interest by directing students to self-appraising activities. Therefore, what I appreciate most is not the fancy equipment, but the way we use it. We are taught how to learn, we are stimulated to evolve individually and to create a personalised study plan that will suit our needs. The innovative spirit is what I love the most about my medical school.

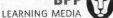

What I hate about medical school

Perhaps my fresher's enthusiasm has partially blinded me, for I find it very difficult to decide what I dislike about the medical school. I can honestly say there is nothing I absolutely hate, but at times I find ranking quite distressing. Unlike many other medical schools, the University of St Andrews ranks all the medics according to their results. This ranking is necessary for deciding the distribution of the students to their chosen universities for the clinical years; therefore ranking stops as soon as the allocation is done. This process can be beneficial, as it stimulates students to study harder in order to reach the desired class position. On the other hand, the rank is not always the desired one and this can become very upsetting. All in all, even though I find ranking quite painful, I think in the long run it will have a positive effect and it will enable me to adopt a fair competition spirit.

Most valuable experience

I shall never forget my first day in the Dissection Room. Having been in the medical school for only a week, the DR was an exciting thought for all of us. The two hours spent examining the allocated body changed my whole perception on life, death and moral values. I suddenly realised how lucky I am to benefit from such a wonderful educational tool. Those courageous people proved their gratitude by donating their bodies, and this is why they deserve our consideration, confidentiality and appreciation. Perhaps that early experience did not offer much scientific knowledge, but it made me realise that a good doctor is much more that a problem-solver. A good doctor respects the patient unconditionally.

Least valuable experience

I have spent hours thinking about my least valuable experience and yet I did not reach a conclusion. Being a fresher, I barely had the chance to adapt to the new environment. Everything seems so new that each experience is unique, interesting and worthwhile. Of course, there will always be dull lectures, less exciting guided studies or even e-portfolio tasks that, for the moment, make no sense. But none of them should be overlooked. I am aware that each experience is there to prepare me for my future job; therefore all of them have a value that will become apparent sooner or later.

The future

My training in medicine has only begun, but I am sure there's a bright career ahead of me. Despite the financial crisis, the EWTD (European Working Time Directive) and the new pension legislation, I am not distressed about the future. On the contrary, I feel reassured that I have chosen the right pathway in life. I do not have regrets or

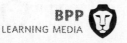

disappointments and I am convinced that everyone feels the same as long as they chose this degree out of passion. By sharing my personal experiences I want to help the readers understand that medicine implies a lot of effort and work, but it can also be fun and rewarding. Never let difficulties overcome you on your way to success!

Ten things I wish I had known before starting medical school

1. Members of staff are there to help you and answer your questions.

2. Study groups can be very beneficial.

3. You should not be afraid to try new methods of learning.

4. Practising clinical skills regularly is a must.

5. Older students can be the best guides. Don't be afraid to ask them anything!

6. Time is short and studies pile up quickly. Never leave things to the last moment.

7. There is always too little time during reading week. Studies never go as planned.

8. OSCE and OSPE are not difficult. Just pace yourself.

9. Medical school is fun. You are there to enjoy it.

10. You study for yourself, not for your exams!

Practical Guidance Tips

Application process:

- The format of your personal statement is not important. Just make sure you write down all your valuable experiences.

- Do not hesitate to read preparatory books for your exams / interviews. They are a lot more helpful than they may initially seem.

- The UKCAT / BMAT play a vital role in the application process. Take your time to properly read and work for these exams.

- Interviews are not as difficult as they seem, but you need to keep calm. Think through your answers before talking and do not be ashamed to pause if you need to.

- The interviewers are not mean or frightening. If they seem so, they might play the 'good cop / bad cop' game. Do not feel intimidated by them.

- If things don't go the way you planned, learn from your mistakes and move on. You will have success in the end!

In medical school:

- Do not let studies pile up. Learn everything as you go.

- Complete the e-portfolio tasks within the deadline. This way you don't have to worry about it the night before your OSCE.

- Go to lectures. Even if they are early in the morning. The handout is not sufficient most of the time.

- Participate in a few societies. It will help you with your studies and social life, and it will look great on your CV.

- Go out and have fun. You do not want to overload yourself.

> 'Think about the hardest you have ever worked previously, then quadruple it – that is the commitment required'

Name: Nina Shavel
Age: 27
University: University of Cambridge
Course: Four-year accelerated graduate course
Year: 1

I originally started out wanting to be a research scientist and so after school I applied to Cambridge to read Natural Sciences (Biological). I really enjoyed my course and after undertaking several research projects over the holidays, I decided to start a PhD on cancer cell movement. Unfortunately, personal circumstances prevented me from carrying on with it, so I got a job in medical communications, running conferences and educational programmes for doctors. I found that while I enjoyed research, I truly loved meeting people from different backgrounds and the intellectual challenges of working on a variety of therapeutic areas, learning both the clinical aspects and basic science, which has led me to consider medicine.

I have decided to share my experiences of being a medical student in this book because I believe that it is really important to understand the realities of medical training and I hope that this article can help prospective medical students do just that.

How it all started

I first thought about going into medicine back when I was doing my Natural Sciences degree but at that stage I was much more involved in research and I had little experience of how rewarding the clinical aspects of the sciences I was studying can be. Later on, when I worked in medical communications, I really started to appreciate medicine as a vocation and to see how science, communication skills and dedication to helping people are combined in this career, which was truly attractive to me. It was hard to leave the world of employment to become a full-time student again but I knew that it was the right thing to do and that I wanted medicine to be my lifelong career. This resolution was further confirmed through the work experience I did, including shadowing in A&E and volunteering on hospital wards and at a hospice.

I knew that medical training would be hard work and that it would be the centre of my life for a long time. I understood that at times I would be sleep-deprived and frustrated based on the stories the foundation doctors at A&E had told me, and I knew that I was letting myself in for a long haul of repeated cycles of training, exams and assessments. However, I also expected it to be very rewarding to be able to use the skills I have developed to help people and to make a difference in my own way.

Application

Considering my age and previous degree, I decided to go for an accelerated four-year course. I applied to Oxford and Cambridge, as both offered medical degrees that provide a solid scientific base for the practice of medicine. I also applied to Southampton because it offered a course that was very much inclined towards offering clinical experience from the start.

I found the application process quite stressful, as I did not have much time available. Preparing for the UKCAT was challenging, as the amount of practice material on offer was very limited and the preparation books varied widely. The test also seemed to be just another hoop to jump through despite having a good previous degree.

I was offered a place at Southampton and invited to an interview at Cambridge. The preparation for the interview was challenging, as there was so much to cover – thinking about answers to typical questions, reading medical and NHS news and relevant books, reviewing key GMC guidance, learning about medical ethics etc. I also had not been interviewed for a very long time, so I asked a friend who was in surgical training to go over a few techniques and typical questions with me.

On the day of my interview I was wracked with nerves, as I knew I wanted to study Medicine at Cambridge more than anything. In the first part of the interview I was asked to read a clinical case and an ethical scenario and then invited to the next room where four interviewers were waiting (being interviewed by that many people can be quite daunting). Each interviewer took their turn asking general questions on my personal statement, as well as questions on the material I had just read. I walked out not knowing how well I had done but luckily I got my letter of acceptance for Cambridge very quickly. I was literally jumping with joy, and I felt so lucky and privileged to be offered this opportunity.

The application process in general was challenging at times, especially because of my other commitments. While I think the UKCAT is not a good way of assessing graduate aptitude for Medicine, I feel that the interviews are absolutely necessary because they are the only way that the university can integrate their personal experience of you with a formal application form to assess whether you would make a good doctor.

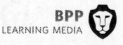

Life as a first year medical student

Typical day

I tend to get up around 7.30am to get to the centre of Cambridge for my 9.00am lectures. Generally I am busy from 9.00am to 1.00pm with a mixture of lectures and practicals followed by supervisions or further practicals on most afternoons. When I get back (around 5.00 – 6.30pm), I tend to review tomorrow's material before dinner. As I prefer not to work in the evenings, I choose to leave them free and use weekends to catch up on the work.

Workload

My average week includes ten lectures, four supervisions (small group teaching) and six to eight hours of practicals (including four hours of dissection work). My free time is all in the evenings (around 20 hours a week), as I tend to study during the day and on weekends (around 25 – 35 hours a week). As the Cambridge course covers anatomy very fast and has a relatively high number of scheduled sessions, I do feel quite overwhelmed by the amount of work (particularly anatomy), especially because, unlike the undergraduates, my holidays are very short. Prioritising supervision material and assignments is very important, as it can be done in the time available and it ensures that you cover key aspects of the work for that week.

Assessments

On a weekly basis we tend to get multiple choice questions (MCQs) or an assignment in each subject which are assessed by the supervisors as the basis for a progress report to your Director of Studies. We also have a college mock exam in January, which is also used to assess progress.

At the end of Year 1, we have first year examinations on the following subjects: anatomy, physiology, molecular biology / biochemistry, medical sociology (essays) and epidemiology / medical statistics (MCQs). The first three subjects are assessed by MCQs on theory, as well as practical examinations. I believe the assessments above are fair, as everything you need to know is covered on the course, and as doctors we do need a good grounding in these sciences. The only difficult aspect is that at Cambridge you are required to know the precise origin and attachment of the muscles, which increases the workload for anatomy.

Social life

I tend to go out in the evening around once or twice a week, mostly on weekends, as during the week I can get quite tired. My husband

and I also like to invite people over to our flat, and I regularly meet up with friends in our favourite coffee shop in town as well. My social circle consists only of medics (and their partners), which is quite an easy habit to fall into, as all of you have similar concerns and experiences.

I think my social life is affected more during the week, when I may not have as much energy, but I do everything I used to do before at the weekend. It is not really about time management for me personally, more about not being motivated to go into town on weekday evenings.

I wanted to take up rowing when I started the course but getting up at 6.30am turned out to be very difficult. I also tend to use the extra half an hour before 9.00am lectures for revision or lecture preparation, which does not fit into the rowing schedule. So instead of formal sport commitments I choose to go running and to the gym whenever I can fit that in, as it helps keep me sane and provides a bit of physical work to balance all the mental effort.

Expectations versus reality

I always knew that medical school would be hard work but I was still blindsided a little by the anatomy workload. Having four hours of dissection work a week can be difficult, especially if you do not enjoy it, and the resulting mass of information requires a significant amount of work. I haven't needed to revise material as I went along previously but with anatomy it is very important.

On the clinical placement side the teaching is pretty much as I expected, although the standard of accommodation can vary a lot. At the moment most nights I drive home after the hospital day is done to get a break and sleep in a nicer environment. I did not expect great accommodation, as it is the NHS after all, but I am used to having my own place and I find it that it is much more conducive to work and relaxation.

What I love about medical school

I love observing doctors helping patients and participating in this process to the extent of my currently limited abilities. On my last placement I found the consultation process in a diabetes clinic fascinating in seeing how different patients relate to their condition and how it can affect their control. It was wonderful to encounter older patients who are living a full life with type 1 diabetes when you think that before insulin the majority died before 20 years of age. Cases like this are a testament to what medical research can do and they inspire me to think about becoming a clinician scientist.

The amazing complexity of human beings means that the consultation process and the management of patients are never truly simple or

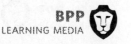

fully worked out. The patience, understanding and empathy that doctors need to have is apparent when you observe their interactions with patients. In chronic disease in particular, the doctor needs to use their communication skills to motivate the patient and establish a mutually agreed plan, as it is often the patient who has to work to improve their health day-to-day. I love the challenge of this process because if I can gain these skills the patients' health would truly benefit.

In a different setting I saw how grateful patients can be after an operation to correct a truly disabling condition and even just for the hope that the surgeon can give them. It is inspiring to see patients return to normality in their lives, and it is wonderful to see the difference that just being able to carry out daily tasks independently can make.

I love learning about the different medical conditions and how I may be able to help people in the future. Learning the basic science may not be to everyone's taste but I find it truly interesting, partly because I believe that to understand and carry out the research on new medications you need to have a good grasp of the underlying pathways.

What I hate about medical school

I don't find dissections particularly enjoyable, and there are far too many hours timetabled for these sessions every week. I do not feel sick or upset about dissections (mainly because I avoid thinking about them too much) but in my mind, after the first couple of sessions, there is nothing that cannot be learned much more efficiently from prosections. I understand the importance of anatomy but I find that getting to the underlying structures on the subject wastes a lot of time without teaching me much.

As I have done a science degree in the past and the standard experiments are often repeated, I am sometimes frustrated with having to do these again, especially because time is so precious with my current workload. Because of the required attendance target I still have to go to the repeated practical sessions but I believe my time can be much better used going over new material.

Finally, I wish I could be closer to home on my clinical placements because it is important to me to spend time with my husband. At the moment it takes me around an hour and a half a day, which is not too bad, but I know that future placements can be much further, requiring two and a half to three hours of travel every day. This amount of travelling time would be quite tiring for me, especially on long placements, so the choice between highly variable and soulless NHS accommodation and the exhausting drive home will be difficult.

Most valuable experience

I went on a home visit with one of the GPs at my practice recently, visiting an elderly lady at a nursing home who was suffering from melena. Following an examination and a review of her file, we knew that the symptoms may be related to a tumour and further investigation was needed. However, the patient did not have capacity for informed consent due to her dementia and her family made it clear that they did not want any investigations or treatment. It was quite hard to realise that all we could do was treat the symptoms and prescribe end-of-life drugs in this situation, as it goes against your instinct to do your best to help by finding and treating the underlying cause. However, I learned that relieving someone's pain and allowing them to go peacefully at that time in their lives is incredibly valuable in its own right. This case has also given me a new appreciation of how important palliative care is and an admiration for the doctors and nurses who work very hard to make their patients as comfortable as possible.

Least valuable experience

The least valuable session so far was a dissection in which we spent most of the time getting to the underlying structures through subcutaneous fat. I will spare you the full description but it was a long and frankly unpleasant process and I did not learn anything about anatomy during it. However, I did learn that thinking about the actual practical tasks and not about the fact that you are cutting into a subject who was once alive is absolutely crucial in handling dissection well. It is a good lesson in remaining impartial, which is very important for a doctor when you may be dealing with death and suffering every day. We need to empathise with our patients but remain impartial, which is a balance that is hard to achieve and maintain but it is a crucial skill if you want to avoid emotional burnout.

The future

I am not sure what the future holds for me at the moment because I have not accumulated enough clinical experience in different specialties yet. I am really excited about my future rotations in different departments because of the opportunities for such varied experiences. Another aspect that I love about medical training is that once I obtain the necessary skills I can help my patients and see the difference I made in someone else's life. I am also very interested in continuing professional development because I think that acquiring new knowledge and the diversity of human beings will make my medical career truly fascinating. On the other hand, the mountains of paperwork doctors deal with and the never-ending application processes may prove rather frustrating.

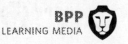

I am too early on in my career to have any true frustrations but I do sometimes worry about the impact of my job on my personal life, although my husband is being incredibly supportive. I hope I will find a specialty that I really love that will allow me to have a balanced life as well. I know that it will not be easy but I did not choose medicine to take the easy path, and I still truly believe that it was the right choice. Hopefully in ten years' time I will be well on my way to the top of my training path and combining clinical work with research in my chosen field.

I hope that you, the new generation of medical students, will find this article helpful and balanced in describing the challenges and rewards of medical training. Read our stories and make sure that medicine is what you truly want to do – it will be hard work but if you know it is right, it will all be worth it!

Ten things I wish I had known before starting medical school

1. Before you decide to apply and certainly before you take up your place, pick up an anatomy textbook and have a very good look. Prepare some material if you can before starting the course.

2. When preparing for interviews and for the application in general, talk to a doctor in training – they can provide valuable advice and a realistic perspective.

3. You will work very hard but make sure that you balance it with other commitments, eg sport, social life, hobbies, as this will keep you sane.

4. Make sure you can cope with learning about the fragility of the human body every day.

5. Volunteer at a hospice – you need to know you can deal with death.

6. Feeling behind is completely normal, it is not just you!

7. Get a good support network – it absolutely crucial when you feel overwhelmed.

8. Be prepared for medicine to be the centre of your life but try to take an occasional day off with a ban on studying or medical talk.

9. NHS accommodation is nothing like home and the standards vary a huge amount, be prepared for mould, strange smells…

10. Think about the hardest you have ever worked previously, then quadruple it – that is the commitment required.

Practical Guidance Tips

- Practise for your interview with someone who is still in medical training because they get interviewed frequently and they learn a huge amount from their experiences.

- Review what you have learned regularly, particularly anatomy – this will make preparing for exams much easier.

BPP
LEARNING MEDIA

'Seeing a birth was something I was particularly excited about, even before starting medical school, so being able to actually assist with one so early on was fantastic. It truly is a beautiful thing to be part of.'

Name: Ruth Collins
Age: 26
University: Swansea University
Course: Four-year accelerated graduate entry medicine programme
Year: 1
Extra info: Masters in Research Methods

Initially I read Psychology at undergraduate level and was convinced that I was destined to be a Clinical Psychologist. In retrospect I think my desire to pursue Clinical Psychology was probably driven by a belief that this was the closest career to medicine I could achieve given the path I'd chosen. After graduating I worked part-time as a researcher while studying part time for a masters in Research Methods. I remember at the time not being particularly excited by the material of my course although at the time I think I saw it simply as a stepping stone. Comparing it to my course now however it seems incredible that I followed that path for so long. I can't imagine working in that area anymore. Until two years ago I was unaware that graduate medical courses existed and I am keen to give potential applicants a brief insight into graduate entry courses and what they might expect both throughout the application process and beyond.

How it all started

According to my parents, I was sure I wanted to be a surgeon from childhood. When it came to making A level choices however, I failed to select the prerequisite science modules. Despite having an interest in this area I think fundamentally I was lacking the confidence in myself and my abilities to see a career in medicine as an attainable goal: medicine had always seemed to me as an option open only to the very gifted. It was not until much later that I came to realise how incredibly normal many doctors are. That is not to say they are unintelligent, but I have come to understand that what stands most successful medical applicants apart is not their mental aptitude but instead their motivation and dedication to their work.

When it came to making selections for A level I think I simply chose what I enjoyed at the time. I honestly had no idea about the type of careers a degree in Psychology lead to. I remember sitting down with a particularly unenthused careers adviser and not once being asked to think about what I actually wanted to do as a career. It was not until my third year that I even began to consider what area I wanted to work in. My experience of working in research and the field of Clinical Psychology however left me feeling frustrated. I was excited by the prospects of working with patients when the research was completed I felt like I was letting the patients down. This was especially the case in clinical psychology where the cohorts we were studying wanted answers and to be directed to local services which often didn't exist. While I could see the benefit of such work, the application was not tangible enough for me. I wanted to be part of something with immediate consequences, where I felt I was really making a positive difference. When I learnt about graduate entry medical courses it seemed like a very natural choice to apply. Working as a research assistant wasn't all negative though. As well as giving me a vital insight into the dynamic and exciting world of medicine, it had also provided me with the confidence and self belief to try.

Application

Having neither a science based degree nor the required A level subjects; I was somewhat restricted in my eligibility for application to many courses. Fortunately, not all institutions were as particular on eligibility criteria. I applied in two consecutive years, mainly to London universities as my life was based there but also to some institutions which were further afield, succeeding in my second application. The most applicable words I could use to describe the application procedure are 'emotional rollercoaster'. I recall the GAMSAT as a particularly strange experience both in the scale of the examination and the behaviours of the individuals taking the exam. I remember for instance some participants popping caffeine tablets and administering eye drops throughout the examination. I remember turning up for the exams literally thinking the rest of my life was being decided that day. After my first attempt I was convinced I would never put myself through the experience again. After a little time to reflect on what had gone wrong however, I did choose to reapply and have never looked back.

The interview process lasted a full day, starting with a talk from the Dean of Medicine, listing the features of the medical school. I remember talking to several people and mentally assessing their backgrounds and experience against mine – something I did not fare well in as far as I was concerned (and something I would not encourage others to do). The talk was followed by a tour of the school and lunch where I inadvertently made a friend. As both our interviews were scheduled for later in the day we both began to get increasingly nervous and ended up performing mock interviews on each other. If you'd have told me

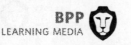

I'd have been doing this the day before or even in the morning I would have never have believed you. Fortunately we were both successful.

The interview itself was both stressful and confusing in equal measure. This being my first medical school interview and having never experienced a good cop / bad cop interview approach before, I left feeling dejected and unsure of the quality of my answers – something which I was later told is the purpose. I remembered particularly having to admit that I didn't know what a word meant and feeling I must definitely have messed it up. The wait seemed to last an eternity. I think to this day I am still unsure of what exactly they are looking for as everyone's interview seems different.

I think probably the single most helpful thing I did to prepare for the interview was to sit down with a colleague, friend, and family, anyone willing to give up their time, to have mock interviews. I found this really helped me formulate succinct and cohesive answers in an eloquent fashion. I think generally while I knew how I wanted to answer most questions often the real life application of this is completely different.

Life as a first year medical student

Teaching days are typically 9.00am through to 5.00pm. This is normally a combination of lecture series and more interactive tutorials in smaller groups based on a 'case of the week' which may be anything from pneumonia to suicide and self harm. Core medical knowledge such as physiology, anatomy, microbiology and pharmacology are taught around this. The integrative nature of the course differs from many of the undergraduate medical courses. Importantly, this method of teaching will not suit everyone as it is dependent on a great deal of self-directed learning, but for me it's a good fit.

Swansea is fairly dynamic in the course design and combines teaching with clinical experience from the outset including community GP placements and a minimum of ten self-selected clinical half days in a specialty of your choosing (although the more enthusiastic students may do as many as they are able). For instance so far, 17 weeks into my medical training, I have scrubbed in on a caesarean section and attended a post mortem as well as self harm assessment interviews and maxillofacial surgery. These placements are a great way of learning more about an area of interest as well as reinforcing the clinical knowledge from previous learning weeks.

The workload is manageable but intense. Given my non-science background I am dependent on my evenings and weekends to brush up on a lot of the science and anatomy; presumably this burden is less for those who have graduated from science or medically oriented disciplines. As well as the volume of work, another way in which the degree differs significantly from my previous degrees is in the mode of assessment. Medical exams are the most nerve-wracking exams I have ever sat. Paradoxically they are also the most fun. Being able to interact with people, interpret clinical data and identify anatomical features beats writing essays any day in my opinion. Swansea also has a great system of transparency in relation to the examination process, feeding back to students what the cohort struggled with to encourage further learning.

Social life

Managing a social life with the demands of the course is difficult but definitely not impossible. I think you will always feel like there is something that needs to be done whether it's writing up your notes, practising clinical skills, revising, or pre-reading in preparation for the week ahead. I try to do something social a couple of times a week outside of the time we spend together at university or on placements even if it's simply watching a movie with friends or a quick drink in the pub. I also try, as much as possible, to leave most of my weekends free to relax. Taking time to relax and switch off is so important to maintain a sense of normality outside of the medical world, which does seem at times all consuming. I think if it weren't for this I would burn out very quickly. Ultimately your free time depends on your time management skills and ability to focus without distractions to ensure you stay on top of the workload. These are skills I have yet to perfect.

Expectations versus reality

The course has far exceeded any expectations I had of medical school. I always knew I would love the application of medicine but I have surprised even myself in how much I love learning about the finer details such as cellular biology, embryology and physiology. I think perhaps in previous degrees I had forgotten what learning should feel like and how enjoyable and passionate you should be about the subject you read.

I think generally I was pretty well prepared for the course in terms of what to expect – probably owing to working in a team of medics and surgeons in my last research job. One thing that did surprise me about medicine however is the all encompassing nature of training. What I was perhaps naive to before starting my education was that the accumulation of knowledge represents just one facet of medical education. In addition to this there are a multitude of skills which need to be learned and honed. This includes development of communication and diagnostic abilities but also mastery of our interpretative skills – ie to understand what *feels*, *sounds*, and *looks* normal. In retrospect I think my view of medical teaching was a little antiquated. The emphasis on varied

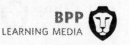
BPP
LEARNING MEDIA

teaching approaches and interactive learning is far more contemporary and completely different to how I had envisioned it on my first few days.

What I love about medical school

The clinical placements are probably the biggest highlight for me so far. In our first year we are expected to complete ten, the only stipulation being that one must be based in a medical specialty, one in surgery and one in psychiatry. The varied nature of these adds such diversity to the term. My favourite placement so far is probably assisting with a caesarean section. Seeing a birth was something I was particularly excited about, even before starting medical school, so being able to actually assist with one so early on was fantastic. It truly is a beautiful thing to be part of.

I've also loved our community based learning placements in local GP surgeries. It still surprises me how open and accommodating patients can be in enabling my learning even when discussing quite intimate problems or concerns. This definitely reinforces for me what a privileged position medical students and the medical profession in general hold. Aside from the clinical placements, the teaching itself is also really great, especially clinical skills. We are fortunate to have some incredible tutors who make the process interactive, dynamic and fun although it did feel quite strange initially talking the examination through to a plastic model. These sessions really give you a chance to familiarise yourself with the techniques but also the associated patient communication. I don't think I realised truly how valuable this was until I was given a chance to practise explaining the details of more intimate examinations during obstetrics and gynaecology week.

What I hate about medical school

There is not as yet anything I could say I hate about medical school but there are certainly things which I have found more challenging than others. For example, our cohort is, from what I hear, quite laid back relative to other schools but the competitive nature of medicine still surprises me several months in. Also, the volume of information is enormous and much of the learning, especially of anatomical knowledge, is by rote. This can be very tedious and time consuming. There are things which do help me personally such as using the anatomy models and working in small groups but for the most part there is not a lot you can do about this. Fortunately, much of the learning will facilitate future learning. For instance, learning the gross anatomy of the bone may aid your understanding of muscle groups and their attachments later. The one thing I think I struggle with the most is constantly staying motivated. In my previous degrees I was lucky in that I only needed to stay focused for short periods at a time around the exams. Studying medicine feels like that all the time. It is quite hard to maintain that level of motivation day in day out.

Most valuable experience

One of the most valuable aspects of the course, aside from the clinical experience we gain on our placements, is the opportunity to talk frankly with patients who have the conditions about which we are learning. This is often a very moving experience and gives us an invaluable insight into the impact of living with these diseases and the practicality of managing your life around them. Often, when learning about different pathologies it is tempting to see patients as a collection of symptoms and clinical signs. I find these sessions really allow us to understand the concerns of the patients and what it means to live with a condition day-to-day. Hopefully this understanding will factor into our clinical decision-making later on.

Least valuable experience

I can honestly say that as yet there are no experiences which strike me as being least valuable. Perhaps this is because I am so early on in my training, or perhaps it stems from entering medical school as a graduate student. I think there is almost always something to learn from most experiences, be they positive or negative. For instance, even situations where you disagree with an approach taken by teachers or clinicians may serve a valuable lesson in guiding the values you hope to represent (or not represent for that matter) once qualified.

The future

Studying medicine as a graduate has both pros and cons to it but one significant aspect as a female is juggling having a family with your medical career, especially as I am starting almost a decade later than most. Certainly one regret is not having had the courage and self belief to have followed this path earlier. Having said that many people manage to balance the two very effectively and training is certainly more flexible now than it has been in the past.

I am still very early on in my training and think I still barely feel like a medical student, let alone a trainee doctor. I am still uncertain as to which specialty I wish to pursue, I think I'm finding it hard to look past each term at the moment let alone attempt to make a plan for the next four years.

I am however attempting to narrow down this process instead by ruling out areas I feel I am not interested in. The problem with this approach, which I think is probably shared by many medical students, is that I find most aspects of medicine fascinating – why else would I be studying it? I'm hoping the clinical placements will give me a better understanding of each specialty and guide this decision although I have a long way to go before one needs to be made (thankfully). What is clear to me however since starting the course is how important the work-life balance is to me

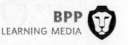

and so I imagine this will factor prominently into my decision of what specialty to follow.

My decision to study medicine, to completely alter my career path, to move to a different country, places an enormous strain on my relationship and will add another few zeros to my already substantial student debt. It was not one I made lightly. Half way through my first year of medical training I have never worked so hard and been so entirely challenged in every conceivable way but I wouldn't change my decision to study for anything. I have also never been so fulfilled.

Ten things I wish I had known before starting medical school

1. Studying medicine is the most fulfilling course I think there is.

2. Be prepared to work harder than you have ever done in your life.

3. The difficulty lies not in the complexity of the work but in the volume.

4. You cannot possibly know everything.

5. Half the battle is learning how you learn best.

6. Be prepared to become intimately comfortable with your body and your classmates' during clinical skills sessions.

7. Have the courage to say no if you do not feel comfortable with what you are being asked to do.

8. Make sure you make time to relax and **not** think about medicine.

9. Bring rubbish clothes to wear for anatomy days – formaldehyde smells awful!

10. Always tell people where you are in your training, especially at the start. It means people won't have ridiculous expectations of you.

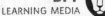

Practical Guidance Tips

- Try not to get caught up in how other people are doing, just do what works for you, after all, you were all smart enough to get a place on the course.

- Make sure you have a good network of friends and family for support, you will probably need to lean on them from time to time.

Chapter 2

The second year: A dose of reality from five medical students

Gareth Wilson

Sana ullah Khan

Michael Hale

John Shenouda

Michael William Mather

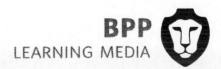

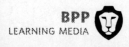

The second year: A dose of reality from five medical students

> 'Don't become a doctor for the status, and certainly don't do it for the money. Do it because you love the subject, and because you love people.'

Name: Gareth Wilson
Age: 25
University: Kings College London
Course: Five-year course (plus one conversion year – no longer done at KCL)
Year: 2
Extra info: Massive football fan

Hi, I'm a second year medical student at GKT. I'm a graduate, but I'm on the traditional five-year course. If all goes to plan, then I'll be graduating in 2014, aged 29. My first degree was French with English, which couldn't be more different from studying medicine, and yet I'd be lying if I said that the study skills my degree taught me weren't transferrable to this course. I'm definitely not a typical medical student, and excluding the fact that I didn't study a science course at university, I also don't have any science A levels, and upon commencement of the course, I had last done GCSE science *seven years ago*.

How it all started

So *how* on earth did I get into medicine, why, and how am I coping, are the questions you may be asking right now. It all started in my second year of university. I had come from a typical grammar school background, where I was expected to go to university, but without any real career aspirations, I simply chose to study the subjects I enjoyed the most. I figured that if I did well enough, then surely work would come later (this is a dangerous assumption in today's job market by the way). I also knew I had a strong desire to help people. This may sound familiar to some of you. In my second year, I ended up volunteering with a homeless charity; I had become sick of walking past the homeless and not doing anything, or simply giving them a bashful smile as I sped along my way. So I decided to help in the only way I could – giving out food, talking to them, trying to coax them into support programmes, and so on. It was an incredibly rewarding experience, and that's all it ever would have been, until I met one man in particular who changed my life. This man had

 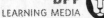

been living on the streets for decades, was a delusional schizophrenic, and was addicted to crystal meth. As he spoke to me all I could think of were his illnesses – he was coughing blood in front of me, all his teeth were missing, he was covered in sores. He was so ill, and I realised all I wanted to do was to fix him. The sense of satisfaction I'd felt at giving out food was replaced with a feeling of inadequacy, the realisation that what I was doing to help just wasn't enough for me, and that I wanted to do more. That led me to considering a career in healthcare.

Medicine wasn't my automatic interest – it was actually nursing. My mother was a nurse, and I was intimately familiar with the amazing work that they do. However, I also craved an intellectual challenge, and I felt I'd be frustrated by not having as much control over patient care as I wanted. I also considered pursuing a career as a paramedic, having been inspired by the paramedics I'd met and by shows on TV(!). However, I ultimately chose medicine because of the unique position that a doctor has in healthcare. The career is demanding, with almost limitless career pathways, and I was attracted to the idea of having a vast array of knowledge and skills at my disposal, and then be able to use them to benefit someone's life.

Application

When I eventually applied for medical school, I applied to the universities that ran courses specifically for people from non-scientific backgrounds. They each offered a foundation year, where two years of science were crammed into one intense year to get us up to speed with the main cohort. On completion, you joined the traditional five-year course the next year. As a result, the interview process, UKCAT scores and requirements were exactly the same, and all foundation students were interviewed in the same group as the traditional course. Since there were only six or so med schools that did this, I chose my favourite four: GKT, Cardiff, Dundee, and Manchester. I was fortunate enough to get interviews from all of them, and as a result had four incredibly diverse interview experiences. The joy of getting an interview rapidly passes however, when you realise how much preparation there is to do; being up to date on NHS politics, the current system of medical training, interesting recent medical developments, and so on. I bought books, and went on forums where people would post the questions they'd been asked. I practised interview technique with friends, and examined and analysed my experiences obsessively. And after all of that, I was still completely unprepared for my Cardiff interview.

You see, they already know you're smart. They already know you're motivated. The interview is about them examining your personal qualities to see if they can imagine you treating patients in five years' time. At Cardiff, I was subjected to an extremely aggressive examination of my qualities, with questions ranging from demanding why I hadn't become

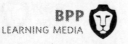

a Taekwondo master in the years I'd been training, to being asked how the brain works. The approach was very much a bad cop / bad cop one, and for about twenty minutes I was verbally battered about the room. Well thought out responses seemed to land on deaf, unimpressed ears, and the interviewers wouldn't deign to look me in the face. I left the room shaken. And yet weeks later, they made me an offer! You see, by pulling me through the wringer, they saw how I coped under pressure, and I guess that must have impressed them (I also like to think my answers hadn't been that bad)!

The interview process is a necessary evil, and I swear many of the people involved get a perverse pleasure out of making the new generation twist in the wind a little. A bit of empathy from admissions departments nationwide would go a long way towards making the process less intense, but I believe it is made this intense for a good reason, because as future doctors, we will all inevitably be under much more severe pressures in our careers. I was fortunate enough to receive four offers in the end, but the feeling of relief you have when you get *any* offer is indescribable.

I had a strong idea of what I'd be letting myself in for in a career in medicine, as I have family members who are doctors, and spent a year working in a hospital after graduation. However, this still doesn't fully prepare one for medical school. You're told it's hard, and that not everyone will make it. But you're also told it's a lot of fun. This is all true. What I didn't realise until getting here though, was that Medicine is a *marathon*. Never underestimate the importance of this fact. I eventually chose Guy's, and now as a 2nd year on the main course, this fact rings true more than ever. A 2nd year medic at GKT can expect to have on average five to six lectures a day, and then have one or two tutorials after that. The year starts off quite slowly, but rapidly picks up pace, and one will spend about seven hours a day at university on the particularly heavy weeks. A typical day will start at 9.00 am 'sharp' (although as jaded 2nd years, this word has been given a somewhat looser interpretation), and lectures will often run in three-hour blocks. All first and second year lectures are held in the Greenwood theatre, a large lecture theatre with seats not designed for the more leggy among us, but at least the walls aren't painted bright orange anymore! We are often only given an hour for lunch, which means you can't wander off too far, or indeed even go home to eat. The lectures are delivered by a wide range of lecturers, although for certain subjects there is some lecturer continuity, and this is highly effective. We have received a lot more clinically orientated lectures this year, which has been pretty much what the entire year has been praying for, as the first year was essentially one long slog through biomedicine. The year group at GKT is alarmingly large; nearly 400 of us in total, and sadly this means that you won't get too meet a large portion of your year group. For me, this year has been typified by numerous encounters with complete strangers in tutorials, or on hospital / GP placements, who although I've never seen them before, have been with me at every step of medical school! It is the most bizarre situation, and a little sad.

Life as a second year medical student

The second year is said to be the joint hardest year of the course, along with the fourth year. We were warned at the start of the year, that without *military* organisation, we would surely be overwhelmed and would fail. This is actually true. Unlike last year, in addition to an increased number of lectures, we are inundated with constant small tests and formative assessments which serve to distract us from the process of keeping on top of the mountain of lectures. For example, in March, we had to complete four or five tests / assessments, which have to be passed in order to even be allowed to take the summer exams. This may not sound like much on paper, but is actually a significant burden that has caused many of my colleagues considerable problems. The quantity of material to learn in the second year is immense and cramming is impossible. You simply have to learn everything as you go along, which can be difficult if you've already spent seven hours of your day studying. But as they say, medicine is an *endurance* sport! Of course, with sufficient self-discipline, the workload is completely manageable. However, it takes the kind of individual who knows how to use their time effectively. You don't need to spend every hour of every day in study; indeed, this is irresponsible and may lead to burnout / insanity. Instead, through organisation and discipline, the second year is hard, but so far, doable.

Social life

As for the work-life balance, this isn't as hard as it sounds! They say that medics work hard and play hard, and this is definitely true. As a 25-year-old graduate, I no longer have any desire to get hammered and hit the clubs every night, but because a medic spends so much time immersed in the world of medicine and study, we take full advantage of our freedom. I play sports, take advantage of the *awesome* diversions that London provides me with, and really value my friends. One of the definite upsides of GKT is the huge range of diversity you'll come across. You see racially, culturally, and nationally diverse groups of friends all hanging together, and it genuinely warms the heart. The younger medics seem to party a lot harder than I did as an undergraduate, and I think this is because we are closeted away from the rest of the university for so much of the day. Our days and terms are longer, our holidays shorter, and so most people (me included) do whatever we can to make up for it.

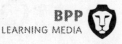

Expectations versus reality

Medical school is almost exactly what I expected it to be, to be honest. I didn't have any particularly romantic notions about the pre-clinical years – just one long hard slog, and that's exactly what it's proven to be. I do have high expectations for next year though, as this is when clinics begin in earnest, and I cannot wait. Anything that gets me out of the lecture theatre and into patient contact is going to be a massive improvement! This makes it sound as if I have hated my time so far, which is completely untrue, however having already completed a four-year degree, I have had my fill of lecture-based learning for now, and am looking forward to getting some hands-on learning under my belt. I said that medical school has held almost no surprises for me, but the one true revelation for me has been the nature of medical learning. GKT runs a traditional, lecture-based course, as opposed to newer problem-based learning courses run at other universities. This has both advantages and disadvantages, but the biggest realisation I have made of pre-clinical medicine, is that it is simply a massive memory test. If you have an incredible memory, you will do well in pre-clinical medicine, as almost no real intelligence or reasoning is needed. Exam questions at Guy's assess one's ability to have retained one tiny detail from the entirety of a lecture. This style of questioning in no way acknowledges or rewards one's understanding of the concept, or knowledge of all other parts of the subject, and this is deeply flawed in my opinion.

What I love about medical school

I feel the best is yet to come from my experience at medical school; the pre-clinical experience is an important grounding for all medical doctors, but I feel the next few years will hold the most enjoyment for me in this course. From what I have done so far though, there have been some truly superb experiences. I can still remember my very first day in the dissection room, and the very first time I made an incision into a cadaver's skin. I remember the first time I held a human heart in my hand, and I will never forget the mixture of horror and fascination on a friend's face as I passed her half of a brain during a neuroanatomy session. There have been so many moments where lifelong curiosities have been answered by knowledge gained on the course, and that has been priceless. I've also really enjoyed living in London. I have never lived here before, and I would recommend anyone to live in a capital city for a time. It is constantly exciting, dynamic, and ever-changing. I have joined hundreds of roller-bladers en masse on the streets of London on a Friday night, darting in between cars and scooters as we 'retake the streets' from the cars for a few hours. I have been to some of the weirdest parts of Camden town and Soho and seen alternative living at its finest, and I have witnessed

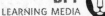

what St Patrick's day celebrations look like in a town where there are more pubs per square mile than anywhere else in the country. Most of all though, my favourite part of medical school so far has been watching how I've grown from my experiences here. I never used to be the type of person who could fill literally every day with activity, who could handle such high workloads, pressure, and still be able to relax, and I am immensely happy that medical school gave me that opportunity to improve myself.

What I hate about medical school

I don't think there's anything that I hate about my time here; sure, I resent the fact that the chair in my room has started to develop depressions in it which happen to share the exact same dimensions of my buttocks, but nothing else really. You come to medical school prepared to work, and there's only so much complaining you can do before you simply have to get on with it! One thing that is very specific to Guy's, and that took me a little while to get used to however, was the feeling of complete anonymity that you have as a medical student. In my opinion, Guy's does not do pastoral care, and you are only ever likely to hear from tutors if you are in trouble for something. A Guy's student will never get to know their lecturers, and will never really feel supported in any way. The stern speeches that we are given at the start of each year firmly espouse the principle of 'sink or swim', which Guy's seems to believe in. Furthermore, the concept of fostering academic competition between students has been strongly encouraged from Year 1. For example, we would receive helpful comments after exam results to show us how well we had done in relation to our peers, and although some individuals may enjoy viewing their colleagues as 'the competition', I and other graduates find this a little tiresome. It adds additional pressure in what is an already high-pressure environment.

Most valuable experience

My biggest challenge so far (save for learning post A level science in four subjects, after a seven year hiatus from science) has simply been learning how to master the work-life balance. After seven hours of lectures (almost a full day's work in the real world), my old reflex was to collapse in front of the TV and relax. No more! The necessity to work, and to use your precious free time for things more edifying than watching 'Neighbours', has driven me into developing a greater level of drive and energy. I feel that I can keep on working, playing sport, or anything I like for longer than I ever thought I could.

Least valuable experience

We are all told that medical school accepts only the best and the brightest (I'm not sure how convinced I am of this, but it *is* good for the ego). The fundamental paradox to this however, is that once you are among similarly brilliant people, your star diminishes somewhat. Many people who go to medical school were among the best in their fields; but when you come here, prepare to feel average. At Guy's, the pass mark for exams is at 50%, with multiple choice questions, and no negative marking. When I heard this I scoffed. How hard can it be to do well? Well, let me put it this way, Guy's, like many other medical schools, has built-in retake sessions in the summer, *in anticipation* of significant numbers failing their exams. If Cambridge graduates, straight-A students, and former pharmacists struggle, then this helps to put things in perspective. Personally, I have found it to be a simultaneously humbling and edifying experience. Medical school can make you doubt your intelligence when nothing else could. However, if you are committed to improvement, you soon realise how to maximise your potential, and become all the better for it. And of course, there are always those people that find everything easy, but we won't talk about them. They're weird.

The future

I really don't think too much about the future at the moment; I have no idea what I want to specialise in, because as a pre-clinical student I haven't really seen anything yet. Nor do I know how far my drive and ambition will take me. My experiences so far have shown me that I enjoy medicine, and that I enjoy the challenges it provides me with. I know that I'm still pretty early on in my medical education, so at the moment I'm keeping an open mind. The clinical years may enthuse me, or may make me re-evaluate what I've been working towards for so long. I simply don't know at the moment. As I've said before, I will be 29 when I qualify (hopefully), and my age, desire to start a family, and other concerns will no doubt have an influence on what I end up doing in my medical career. To paraphrase a wise man, '*the future is always in motion*'.

As yet, I don't feel as if I've made a mistake coming to medical school; even one as impersonal as GKT can be. It has continued to challenge me, to make me grow, to stimulate and entertain me. The life experience that I have gained so far has been truly invaluable, and I hope to continue my adventure in medicine for many years to come. If you're looking at these words and considering a future in medicine, I urge you to take your time and consider your alternatives. It's a marathon, and even once you've qualified, the learning has only just begun. Don't become a doctor for the status, and certainly don't do it for the money. Do it because you love the subject, and because you love people.

 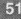

Ten things I wish I had known before starting medical school

1. You don't need to buy any books. Just loan them out from the library.

2. You won't be the best.

3. Gin is not your friend.

4. Your memory is not as good as you think.

5. You really won't see many patients at all in the first two years.

6. Dentists earn more than you.

7. Stay off the coffee until you really need it.

8. Avoid too much red meat (bowel cancer).

9. How important it is to befriend those in the years above you. They know all the tricks.

10. Not to trust London buses.

Practical Guidance Tips

- One of the most important things you can do with your time is properly work out what your most effective learning style is. It is unlikely that your method of staring at the book until the knowledge sinks in will cut it at this level, especially in clinical years, when time is short, and there no revision periods before exams. Take the time to experiment with different learning styles to find what works best for you. It might be mnemonics, spider diagrams, associations... whatever! Just find out – the sooner you do, the easier you'll find med school.

- Make sure you find the time to explore your city. It can be very easy to become lost in a medic's world, one ruled by lectures and timetables. You're already a bit separate from the rest of the uni – make sure you're not separate from the city! You won't regret broadening your horizons.

> *'Anyone who saves one life, it is as if he has saved the whole of mankind and anyone who has killed another person (except in lieu of murder or mischief on earth) it is as if he has killed the whole of mankind.'*
>
> The Holy Quran, Chapter 5, verse 32

Name:	Sana ullah Khan
Age:	23
University:	University of East Anglia
Course:	Five year PBL programme
Year:	2
Extra info:	I love interacting with patients

A little bit about me, well I was born in a city called Peshawar in Pakistan; officially regarded as one of the oldest living cities in Asia. I was exposed to medicine very early, not that I can remember, but I was born very prematurely and as a result my inner ear never developed leaving me congenitally deaf in my left year.

I had a twin sister who unfortunately died 20 years ago and in a country like that; they didn't give my parents much hope for my survival. However, my mother is the single reason why I'm alive today; she nursed me round the clock for months. It's said in my family that she could have easily brought up seven children as opposed to me.

How it all started

I have been fortunate that I was born to a family of highly educated parents. My mother has several degrees while my father is an ENT surgeon.

There are no prizes for guessing what inspired me to want to pick medicine as a career. I'm not one of those people who wanted to study medicine the moment I was born. Growing up, being exposed to my father was one of my motivations. However he didn't really bring his work home with him so I can't say it was that.

I am fairly sure that American sitcoms like Scrubs played a small yet vital role in making that decision; come on, it's not like I'm the only one that thinks like that!

I'll be honest; I come from a South Asian background where in some parts of the culture, they still liken doctors to God. Can I really say it was a mixture of god complex / prestige? I'd slightly subscribe to that. Then

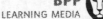 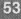

again I think anyone suggesting otherwise is lying or is just in it for all the 'right' reasons.

There's also religion; I'm a practising Muslim, although I'm not totally religious about doing my prayers on time; pun intended. Islam does prescribe a good dose of humanity and goodness to your fellow man; attributes not unlike that of the medical profession.

In short, I can't pinpoint a single reason why I decided to pick medicine but there's also the fact that my mum wanted me to do it!

Life as a second year medical student

The advantage of being on a PBL course is that the weeks make sense, well in theory. We have a modular systems-based course where we study one system at a time. We have a theme of the week and the lectures, seminars and primary care (General Practice) placement all revolve around that theme and in the middle of the module we spend four weeks in hospital.

I'm currently studying respiratory medicine and the previous week's topic title was 'chronic breathlessness'. On Mondays, I have a PBL session from 1.00pm in the afternoon to 3.00pm and then a summary lecture of the previous week. The last bit is really useful if I'm stuck with something from the previous week, and it's given by a clinician, usually a consultant. Tuesdays are packed with seminars from 9.00am until 5.00pm with a lunch break and an hour somewhere in between and Thursdays are the same. There's usually one lecture on Wednesdays, and the rest of the day off. Finally, Friday is the long day at primary care but it's fun.

I might be wrong but I can remember having more lecture hours in college than here at university. This leaves a lot of 'free time' for procrastination (a word you'll pick up at university). However, given the nature of a PBL course, 'free time' equates to time for so-called self-directed learning. That basically means 'there's the library, teach yourself medicine and we (the medical school) will help you along the way'. Its blunt, but it's true. I'm sat here complaining yet ironically I can't see another way of learning medicine. Then there's the workload. It's ridiculous and to be honest I sometimes doubt if it's humanly possible to learn it all, yet somehow there are doctors in this world. No matter how much you try shutting it away; by going out with your mates, going on Facebook or just staring at your books with a blank expression, it's always there, always. I can't pretend to be studious and I can't say how much I study a week but I can tell you how much I should study a week. In theory, I should spend around two hours for every one hour of lecture and more time for revision. I hate swallowing my pride but I'm afraid my dad was right; there's no substitute for hard work; there are no shortcuts in medicine.

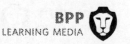

An average medical student's fears are exams and there's a bunch of them. They're ugly no matter what form they come in. There's the portfolio; a once-a-year reflective piece of writing. An analytical review; which consists of analysing a research paper and descriptively writing about it. The Objective Structured Clinical Exams (OSCEs for short); these are more practical and test your clinical skills, reasoning and knowledge; the most fun you can have in an exam. The student selected study (SSS for short; lots of three-letter-acronyms) which is a presentation usually PowerPoint on a topic / field of research. Finally the advanced notice paper (ANP; yes more acronyms); which consists of short answer questions and multiple choice questions. This is the final written exam and it encompasses everything from the year and 25% is based on modules from previous years.

I'm not the biggest fan of exams but they work, I guess. I can't see a way of improving them and really never had a chance to complain about them. Maybe I'll think about it a bit more.

Social life

I really have no describable social life; I try, honestly I do. There are a couple of set nights weekly where the student club on campus holds events and our university really offers an active nightlife. I'm not one to get too excited about clubbing; which is more than can be said about some of my colleagues.

Unfortunately, medics are notorious for drinking and I'm very much in the minority here. I'll be honest; my social life is affected as a result because I'm the odd one that's not 'having fun'. So if you like to drink and would love to be around people that do the same; medical school is a great place to be.

My social life doesn't end because I don't drink, there are lots of social things I do. I cook for friends, go to the cinema or watch movies in my flat with friends, get a take-away and play card games – a little more civilised in my opinion; although it's not to everybody's liking. There are endless social and sports clubs to join at university that hold regular social events; I just don't have the time to fit it all in.

Expectations versus reality

I really had some high expectations about life as a medical student and, I'll be honest, most of them weren't a surprise. I always expected long hours, tedious routines, being overworked and having no social life. I'm glad to report that it's not the case at all, in fact it is a pleasant lifestyle. Sure, you're on your feet a lot of the time, but then again you're on a seat a lot of the time too. I think it's a great way to spend time at university; trust me, it makes time fly.

I admit that most of my non-medical colleagues seem to have a lot of time on their hands and it's clear from their vibrant social life. At least I can take solace in knowing that I'm not the only one in my situation; there are plenty more poor souls in the same boat with me.

It is important however, to read thoroughly about the medical school you decide to apply to. I guarantee that if you don't you'll be disappointed by some aspects of the course; whether it's the teaching or the course style. I can't say what it would be like to study a traditional course; but in my PBL-style course, things make sense to me. We go through the body in systems and our learning encompasses the basic medical sciences like anatomy, physiology, biochemistry etc. We learn all there is to know about that system and see patients with related illnesses during the week and then in secondary care during the module. This style makes sense to me, it agrees with my view of a holistic approach towards patient care.

What I love about medical school

Where do I start? I love the fact that I have a goal to achieve; it really makes a difference. I know it's sad but knowing that at least after medical school you have job security (mostly true) and you'll be a doctor. A doctor; someone who is a highly educated, well-respected functioning member of society; it scares me to think one day soon I will be a doctor.

The nature of the course lends itself to variety; it's nice to be able to switch topics if I'm bored of studying one topic.

A concept known as spiral learning got into my head in med school; it just means that you'll be constantly learning about a topic long after you've finished it. The higher up you go in med school; the more pieces of a jigsaw puzzle you can put together.

The next bit is going to sound really sad but there's nothing like the ecstasy of getting your first diagnosis and then the second and so on. All that reading pays off – you see a patient exhibiting signs and symptoms and it's great to list a differential of all the possible causes and then break it down to that one potential culprit. It's like being a detective; someone comes in with a mystery; you ask them what they know about it which is history taking. You collect all the clues and you come up with a list of suspects in your head. You examine, investigate and confirm your diagnosis. I'm not Sherlock Holmes but it'll be the closest I ever get.

Medicine makes sense most of the time; its findings can be used in real life and even the theories can be used in real-life situations. I doubt that's the case in many other professions; in medicine unless

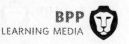

you specialise you need to use nearly everything you know. Its great knowing that at least the reading you're doing will not only benefit you, but also your patients and you can put your knowledge into practice.

The next bit is cheesy and probably not that important but I'll share it anyways. I love the patients I see; they're what make my day. They motivate me to study; they encourage my curiosity and drive my passion; not to forget they're so lovely. In my experience patients are always delighted to see medical students. They've always treated me so well and usually I can see the admiration in their eyes as if to say 'keep trying'. In my experience they treat you like they would treat a doctor but without the fear without the need to hide things and without the hesitation. They're usually so open, honest and willing to share their stories and experiences. It's such a privilege to be able to sit next to a total stranger and have them confide in you; I've had patients tell me things they admit to not telling their loved ones or even their doctors! The patients will have to top my list of things I love about medical school.

What I hate about medical school

There are a number of things that I really dislike about medical school but hate is a strong word especially when there are things I can't change. Imagine being in a class with a couple of hundred other competitive, highly achieving ambitious people; it makes me choke at times. I mean the worst part is when other students pretend they don't work and lie so much about the amount of work they put in. It's infuriating, childish and rather unprofessional; I know it's blunt but I think it's just wrong.

I always imagined medical students as dedicated, passionate, polite individuals who set the trend for other members of society to aspire to achieve; the perfect gentlemen / women if you will. I really don't know why I imagined that; the secret is they're like the rest of the population.

As medical students professionalism is an integral part of our daily life. We are advised by the medical school and to some extent the General Medical Council to show a great image to the public.

Most valuable experience

It's really hard to describe my most valuable experience at medical school. I've learnt a lot about how to organise and prioritise my life.

The most important thing I've learnt in medical school is being true to oneself. I'm still trying but I'll refine it soon enough. A great tool for this is reflection which we will use a lot in our professional careers too. I learnt not to be scared to reflect, criticise and as a result refine my methods. I try to implement this in my whole life rather than just in life as a medical student but it's not easy to admit when I'm wrong. In my experience, it took a few attempts and then after swallowing my pride I'd implement small changes. A small example is acting on feedback from my tutors on my quality of work and sometimes it'd be difficult because criticism isn't something everyone readily takes on board. I started by reflecting on some of the suggested improvements and analysed them to see if they were something I'd happily apply. The result was that sometimes I wouldn't and sometimes I felt my way needed a little refining to suit their requirements; a win-win situation really.

The future

This is a huge question and one that's always shrouded with mystery for me. I hope that within the next ten years I will have graduated medical school and made a steady progress up the long career ladder.

I'm very optimistic about the future of medicine and I hope I can play a little part in the grand scheme. I came to medicine with an open mind so my future specialty is up in the air and I'm hoping a few will entice me in medical school to narrow the options. This is where the structure of my course at UEA comes in handy because as I complete a module I decide if I like it enough to see myself in it in the future. Of course a lot of it depends on the influences it has on me and there are a few that I am interested in.

I tend to consider the scope of a subject; its future and how much it can impact on a patient's quality of life. I also consider research, its pace and the predictions about what its impact will be during my career.

The accelerated pace of technological advancement and research makes me feel privileged to be part of a generation of doctors that will see real development and change in how we battle human suffering. I know it sounds clichéd but no matter how hard the challenges to come will be, there's no doubt that this is the most exciting time to be studying medicine.

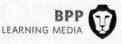

Ten things I wish I had known before starting medical school

1. It would have been handy to be told the reality of what I was about to undertake. Every day I wake up to a mountain of work, housekeeping and social responsibilities.

2. I really wished I had stayed at home – after a long day of ward rounds, coming home to a cupboard with no food can be devastating.

3. I wish someone would have told me how fast I'd grow up. It happens; your priorities change.

4. In medicine, learning is lifelong and not just the five years; bear that in mind.

5. Be prepared to change your views or what you've learnt; medicine changes.

6. You'll have to work harder, longer and better than most of your non-medical flatmates and try not to feel disheartened when they're going out every other night and you can't.

7. Bring an extra couple of bags of motivation and happiness with you.

8. Prepare for the back stabbing, back biting, narcissistic, sarcastic colleagues you'll come across at medical school. They're not that uncommon.

9. Learn to accept criticism with a smile and 'dance to their music'.

10. Medical school will try and change you; don't let it. Stay strong and be the person you are because it's that personality that got you into medical school in the first place.

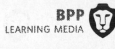

Name: Michael Hale
Age: 24
University: University of Warwick
Course: MbChb five-year course
Year: 2
Extra info: Mature student

As a mature student at Warwick Medical School (WMS) I've embraced life as a 'medic' with open arms having fought hard to get here. With a Biochemistry degree and five applications for Medicine I came from each and every angle, trying all and everything to get into medical school. During my first degree I began to contemplate the wider implications of a career outside of medicine, that inspired nothing at all, further fuelling my desire to apply repeatedly. Now studying a degree I sacrificed so much to get onto I felt it right to share my experiences of the further sacrifices required once that ever elusive place at medical school is finally secured.

How it all started

It all began when I was turned away from a careers talk for medicine due to my GCSE scores. Determined to prove my teachers wrong, I made my first application at 17.

Thinking about what a medical career meant to me without any clinical exposure was difficult. As a teenager unwilling to commit to anything other than rugby six times a week, a career with such diverse opportunities seemed perfect. It was later that I began to contemplate whether or not I could help people, and a few weeks after starting this I had no doubts that this was going to be a rough ride. My disciplinary record at school wasn't great, however a love for people and an aching feeling of loss when I scored miserably in my AS levels was the push I needed.

I have never been pressured by my parents, just urged to behave and encouraged to be the best I could be. My parents always advocate good manners, big smiles and an open mind, something that has driven me to bigger and better things throughout my life.

Application

With five applications it's hard to remember all the places I've applied to, my reasons varied, sometimes I applied because I fancied training in a particular city. Other times I played the numbers game, and the rest of the time I based my choices on the style of the course.

Each application was tough so I used them as learning tools, trying to increase focus, and be stronger and more prepared with each application. The application is neither exciting nor stressful but more insightful with the process allowing you to reflect on what it is you need to do in order to beat the competition.

My first interview at the University of Liverpool involved an in-depth discussion about politics and medicine. Reflecting back immediately afterwards I realised I knew distinctly little about both of these things and would have to rectify that and other things if I truly wanted to be a doctor. A good knowledge of medicine in the real world is essential for any successful interview.

Following this interview I began viewing any interview as a conversation I would have with a family member or friend about medicine, talking in this context brought medicine to real-life and helped me to relate to it as an everyday part of me.

The application process is harsh but fair, and many great applicants will not make it through this rigorous process. The only way to beat the system is to work hard, tick boxes and be committed.

Getting accepted was a really great day, after weeks of reading medical forums and believing all hope to be lost, I had a place.

Life as a second year medical student

This semester my day began just before 6.00am with Radio 4, porridge on toast accompanied by a friend of mine before cycling to university. The cycle clears the head before a full day studying, and luckily for us we had just one road traffic incident. Lectures started at 9.00am with the early start giving me a chance to get on top of things before the day really got going. Lectures are followed by group work involving structured questions linked to the lectures, this is completed with the same group each session. Another lecture finishes the morning session about 12.30, giving us an hour to battle for the microwave or locate a quiet room to squeeze in more work. Afternoon lectures began at 1.45pm and generally had the same format as the morning thus four lectures and two sets of group work each day. Depending whether or not we had evening teaching provided by the year above determined how late I would stay at university, typically I'd try to be home by 9.30pm. Arriving home, I'd devour half a loaf worth of toast and a mug of tea before starting the late shift. This lasted until just after the changeover from Radio 4 to the BBC World Service at 1.00am, fuelling my patriotism with the national anthem most nights before bed.

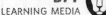

A huge workload to tackle and less than two weeks to revise for our exams – a great deal of my cohort felt the squeeze right from the start of term. I didn't for a minute underestimate the challenge faced, hence the ridiculous daily routine. This obviously varied from person to person but not being academically blessed I felt for me this amount of work was required to perform come exam season (I spent over 100 hours each week studying and did so from week 1). While this isn't ideal, I'm a 2nd year medical student and at times you have to sit tight, ride the wave and hope you can absorb bits as you go while trying desperately to cram the rest of it in before exams.

Three major sets of exams in 12 months has been tough, each involving 20 integrated questions with varying lengths of short answer question. Questions are pass or fail and each question has a different pass mark depending on the performance of your peers. The exams have been extremely controversial but on the whole I feel they're tough but fair, highlighting the importance of lateral thinking under pressure ... as will be required in clinical practice.

Social life

Recently nights out have been few and far between with maybe only two or three notable nights out this semester, all followed by sore heads and the harsh realisation that hung-over study was the only option. A social life has developed which differs greatly from the one to which I had become accustomed during my first degree. The first few semesters at WMS provides ample opportunity for socialising and what appears to be a full timetable at the outset soon has gaps ideally placed to accommodate nights playing beer-pong and getting to know your peers.

Retiring from rugby before starting at WMS was hard for me and I've struggled to find a sport I'm happy to sacrifice study time in order to pursue. I am lucky to have found a group of lads all with same mindset as myself thus we spend a lot of time 'getting massive', competing in various challenges whether that be press-ups, cycling as the 'four winds' (or racing each other to UHCW for placement!), or completing common-room obstacle courses. Any time spent doing exercise allows us to forget medicine for just a short time, an added bonus is getting the blood pumping so your more focused when it comes to studying again.

Expectations versus reality

I didn't expect medicine to be such a bubble, such a concentrated experience where medics and medicine consume your every moment. After six weeks of medical school it hit me hard that I hadn't read the paper or listened to the radio. Following on from that stark realisation I struggled to find ways to expose myself to things non-

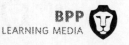

medical – it requires a concerted effort but is terribly rewarding. This realisation helped me appreciate what I had but also what I lacked in my life as a medical student surrounded by medical students.

I always felt medicine would be extremely academically challenging, it isn't. (Well, at times)! Medicine is a test of sleep deprivation, mass movements of information in short periods of time and coping under pressure with people who always, I repeat always, expect more from you than you might expect from yourself.

What I love about medical school

Medical school is hard work and you'll be isolated from the real world with friends who wonder why you don't return their calls or why you said clavicle instead of collarbone. Merely being at medical school makes you different bestowing upon you a responsibility that at times is hard to accept. I have come to appreciate the support network that exists at WMS, the friends I've made, the people I've studied with and those who mentor me day-to-day, they're invaluable and without them I would struggle to cope, well, without copious amounts of coffee.

Medical school can be extremely competitive but in my experience it has been a place where you can never fail to find the answer. While I may have gaps in my knowledge, I can rest assured that one of my peers will be able to enlighten me – this isn't cheating ... just utilising resources. It's a great feeling helping others, and at the end of the day I know things others don't (very occasionally) and by teaching somebody else you reaffirm your knowledge – a win-win situation really. This will become more of a reality in clinical practice when you must utilise anybody and everybody for the benefit of the patient, you will not always know the answer, thus be prepared to be unprepared.

Exposure to patients happened in week 3. While extremely scary it's also vital and visiting patients in their own homes gives a real sense of what you're working towards and the wider implications of healthcare early on in your career as a medical student. Patient contact is priceless, medical students have more freedom and power to roam hospitals than anybody else. I have often found myself lost in hospital and when questioned, the response *'I'm a medical student trying to get a bit more of an idea of what goes on down here...'* is usually met with a smile and extremely helpful explanation, great when you have no idea where you are.

What I hate about medical school

With five attempts to actually get into medical school it is hard for me to find anything to hate, but I'll give it a go.

The 'Medic Bubble' would be the thing I most like and dislike about medical school, you don't know about it until you're six weeks in and well and truly a 'medic'. I'm sure medics across the land hate the medic rumour-mill, an integral part of the 'Medic Bubble'. I'm almost 100% certain someone is employed to spread gossip at WMS; I have my suspicions, but I believe every medical school has the same 'problem'.

I mentioned earlier about the realisation that I lacked exposure to the outside world, for some people that's fine but personally I couldn't quite hack a life solely focused on medicine. Around exam time when you up your game, hit 18-hour study days and dream about drug names and medical models of health you realise there should be more to life. Deal with this by being proactive and break out of that bubble. For me, I joined other clubs, got a job and went home to see old family and friends.

I hate wasted time. Once your studies take full flight and you're squeezing lectures, flashcards, quizzing and the rest of life's essentials into 24 hours you soon develop a real hatred for any time wasted. My time saving tips include... brushing your teeth while showering, doing admin when you're too tired to do real work, fill breaks with productive tasks like lunch making for the next day, get a good hands-free kit and talk to friends when you're cooking or tidying your room, most importantly... sleep when you're tired to save on unproductive tired time.

Most valuable experience

I have two I'd like to mention... cheeky I know.

My first patient case, where I interviewed a blind toddler and her family, was an extremely humbling experience. We had a cup of tea and played with this lovely little girl. We didn't stick rigidly to the framework for structured questioning and learnt so much by watching the family interact in a somewhat awkward semi-social / professional situation. This taught me the importance of putting people at ease to maximise your exposure to them enabling them to relax into meetings with healthcare professionals at any level.

Second, more recently I managed a patient history that was thorough, professional and with good patient rapport, but failed to obtain the patient's name. This is something I'd done under OSCE (Practical Clinical Skills Examinations) conditions in the summer and thought I had learnt from. Realising halfway through I continued until the end of my history before apologising and asking the patients' name (despite knowing it as it was on the board above his bed). My group queried why ask for the patient's name when we were due to read his notes afterwards anyway. It was a matter of principle and common decency; in normal everyday life you'd introduce yourself and ask for someone's name, in hospital

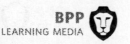

you are dealing with real people. Sometimes it is easy to consider patients as conditions and forget to treat them as people. For me, patient experiences should focus on dealing with patients as people so always remember your manners, as my dad always says 'Manner maketh man'.

Least valuable experience

I came to medical school to learn everything I possibly could to be a good doctor, my learning is least valuable if I don't enjoy it or I'm tired.

I always try to find a way to enjoy my learning environment. If you don't like lectures then try to enjoy the bits around lectures like speaking to your friends; if you concentrate in lectures you can chill after with your mates. If your consultant is rubbish, think well this is better than being stuck in a lecture theatre.

To address tiredness all I can suggest is sleep when you're tired, eat well and try to keep a good well balanced work-life arrangement.

The future

I don't think about my future career as a doctor, preferring to take things one step at a time. I feel that focusing my efforts at one particular specialty too early would be criminal. As a bit of a 'committophobe' in all aspects of my life the idea of another few years without having to go down one particular path is ideal for me. The exciting part of medicine for me is that learning all this material which is clinically applicable will open more doors than I can begin to imagine.

Considering my future aspirations as a doctor, peer approval is a bigger deal than any accolade from the powers that be, thus my aspiration is to be the doctor that people want to refer patients onto within my chosen specialty. I have always felt if your peers think you're good and your patients leave with smiles on their faces, or at least not threatening legal action, then you must be doing something right.

I'd like to do some work abroad and am learning Spanish with the view to use that to travel and work at some point. I would also like to return to a place called Thica in Kenya where I spent some time working with a family health centre. The desolate poverty and lack of doctors means I'd love to go back and offer my services.

I hope to 'make a difference', a sickeningly cliché I know, to as many people as I can. The piece you have just read is an honest account of my journey to a point where I now wake up every single day loving life wondering if I could possibly be doing anything else that would enthuse me so.

 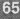

It's been a hard fought battle and I hope this piece makes you think about what you are about to commit to whether it be for the first or fifth time. I quote the motto of a school I visited in Kenya '*Never ever give up*', I feel exactly that for medicine. It is worth the wait, the late nights, the coffee breath, taking a slagging on the rumour mill after one too many last night, worth the money spent on coloured pens and pencils because after all if something is worth having, it is worth working hard for. I unreservedly recommend medicine to anybody interested in a career that knows no boundaries and helps millions of people worldwide every single day.

Ten things I wish I had known before starting medical school

1. Learn big and learn broad.

2. Be prepared to be unprepared.

3. Nurses can be a medical students' best friend.

4. Get good with numbers… it's sort of essential for prescribing.

5. Good sense of smell… lose it or swap it for a good stomach at least.

6. Value your peers… they'll help show you how little you really know.

7. Learn how to learn effectively… this will save your joints from some serious arthritis after countless pages of note taking.

8. If you have a question, ask it. You won't be the only one, just please don't be the loudmouth who pipes up every single lecture.

9. At times you'll sit there, look at your things to do list (mine are often as long as my arm) and feel like all hope is lost… sometimes it is. At these times your non-medic friends will simply not understand why you've so much work, why you can't understand the work you've been given and most often why is it you haven't spoken to them for weeks. No point crying, moaning or swearing (though I'm sure that's been scientifically proven to help, well maybe!), the only thing to do is take a deep breath look at the next item on your list and crack on. Doing anything else isn't getting you any farther down your list, though you could maybe squeeze a cheeky cuppa in just to refocus of course.

10. *Never ever give up.*

Practical Guidance Tips

- Don't just get normal types of experience for your application, do the weird and wonderful to make your application stand out from the crowd!

- Think now about where you might want to end up and start ticking the boxes to get you there… it'll only make things easier later down the line!

> 'Rumour has it that medical students live enclosed lives in dark libraries feeding on ready-made meals and powdered soup. Rest assured, that's only the case pre-exams!'

Name: John Shenouda
Age: 19
University: University of Sussex
Course: Five years
Year: 2
Extra info: I enjoy basketball, tennis and football

Having been through the vigorous application process with all its highs and lows, I thought it only fair to shed some light upon the situation you may currently find yourself in thinking about pursuing a career in medicine. I am an undergraduate student who didn't take a gap year simply because I didn't trust myself with a whole year out of education. I'd much rather delve right into a coveted place at medical school to start, and finish, the long course as soon as possible. And I simply couldn't wait to experience uni life and everything it had to offer from sports to socials and societies; not forgetting the academic side too of course.

How it all started

Clichéd as it may be my desire to become a doctor was a genuine childhood dream, aided by the influence of my parents who just so happened to be doctors. Of course for most people the title, the thought of a life of service and the money seem to be good enough alluring factors. And it must be said, they were for me too. Applying at a time when Britain just hit the economic crisis, it seemed that medicine was one of the very few careers in which you would almost certainly be guaranteed a job and stable income. But the time I actively started thinking about medicine was in Year 11. It hit me that I'd need to be a 'straight A student' to just put me on a level playing field with other applicants. And it was then I began looking into other activities that would put me ahead of the pack.

My older brother was studying medicine and was in his final year when I applied. Watching him talking to my parents in almost a completely different language, the language of medicine, fuelled my desire. I wanted that knowledge. I wanted that respect. I wanted to be able to give my parents that same smile that came from talking to him. And so it was also him who inspired me. What's more, seeing him complete the five years in what seemed no time at all meant the length of the course became less of an issue to me.

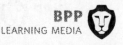

My expectations of medical school were created by all the stories he would tell while at home on weekends. Rarely did he ever break down but when he did, it was almighty. I regularly saw how stressed he was and how much work he had to do. But he still had time to come home every now and again and participate in uni sports as well as having a social life. So although rumour has it that medical students live enclosed lives in dark libraries feeding on ready-made meals and powdered soup, rest assured, that's only the case pre-exams!

Application

I hadn't appreciated the fact that though the application process was essentially still the same, Medicine was much more competitive than it was when my brother applied in 2003. So there was no guaranteeing I'd get in, which again is something I overlooked at the time. I applied to three London universities (Imperial, King's and St George's) as well as one university outside London (Brighton and Sussex Medical School (BSMS)) which was in essence my safety net. Being an active member of my church community at home, I didn't want to move to far away from London to enable me to return at will and be close to my family. As my brother couldn't stop singing London's praises I wanted the chance to live and study in what is one of the greatest cities in the world.

Having spent months trying to sell myself in the application process, the pressure was on. Soon I'd find out whether this was truly my vocation. News of fellow non-medic peers who had received offers from all five of their choices before I'd even heard back from one wasn't reassuring. I got an interview at BSMS in November which was almost like a friendly chat, mostly orientated around my personal statement. (They're not stupid; if you lie on your personal statement, they *will* find out!) This was followed by the first ever OSCE-style interview at George's the same week. I applied to George's knowing that my UKCAT score wasn't brilliant (620) and that they gave interviews based on GCSE results.

With straight rejections from King's and Imperial, George's was later added to that list as the only offer I received was from BSMS. I was delighted I got into medical school but bitterly disappointed that I missed out on a chance to live in London. It was only when I got to BSMS that I realised how fortunate I was to be at the medical school with the highest student satisfaction in the country – and for good reason too.

Life as a second year medical student

A typical day in the life of John Shenouda would go something like the following:

Get to uni for a 9.00am start where we can have between two to four one-hour lectures before lunch at 1.00pm. Then afternoons normally consist of the more hands-on sessions, like dissection or practical imaging classes. These can range in duration from between one and a half hours to three hours long. Finish around 5.00pm then get ready for the evening, be it a sport or a society meeting.

Some key figures for you to digest regarding teaching hours a week:

The average number of lectures a week depends on the module. It's about ten hours weekly and the number of symposia amounts to roughly two hours a week. This excludes practical sessions mentioned earlier which are about four hours weekly. This also excludes Thursdays, our clinical day, where we start with a lecture or two, break off into small discussion groups then go on our clinical placements for the afternoon. All in all you're left with around eight to nine free hours a week (excluding lunch and Wednesday afternoon for sports) which is very reasonable.

The work load is a step up from A levels but it is certainly manageable. BSMS recommend you do around 190 self-directed study hours over the course of the ten-week module. But one must bring to mind that also includes revision time prior to the Knowledge Test (KT) in Week 10 of each module. I personally write up each lecture which takes about an hour. So it works out that for every hour I spend in the lecture theatre, I spend another going over it in my own time. The KT itself consists of SAQs (Short Answer Questions) which often require answers no longer than a paragraph and EMQs (Extended Matching Questions) which are multiple choice questions where you pick an answer from 12 choices.

BSMS has a very student-friendly course structure, with three ten-week terms a year. Each term consists of one systems-based module running alongside the yearly clinical module. There are effectively eight teaching weeks a term with a week or two off at the end to prepare for the KT. The module grade is weighted with the KT contributing 75%. The other 25% is taken up by small assessments such as poster presentations for example. This means over the course of the year, you will have three KTs and one OSCE exam at the end of the year which assesses the clinical aspect.

Social life

Every week I occupy Wednesday to Friday evenings with basketball, tennis and football training for BSMS. Each session lasts two hours excluding matches which vary in frequency depending on the sport. Besides sport, I am a member of the Christian Union, the Medical Society and RAG (Raising and Giving), of which I am President. All three have weekly meetings lasting an hour but RAG takes up considerably more of my time due to the nature of my responsibilities. So in answer

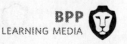

to the question I first asked soon after arriving at medical school... yes! You do have time for a social life; and a pretty good one at that! There's no need for me to explain the night life in Brighton; it's a city renowned for giving students a good time. I just choose to prioritise sport ahead of socials as staying fit is key to my selection for the teams.

There's no denying the sheer quantity of work medics have to do is second to none. But with decent time management, you can have as good a time at uni as any other student on any other course. Besides the typical benefits of sports, they often provide new social circles which aid academically. Students in higher years provide invaluable advice that you can't find in textbooks.

Expectations versus reality

From Week 2 of Term 1 of Year 1, we had been sent out to the wide world of clinical placements. That same week we started our cadaveric dissections; so much for easing you in! On the other hand, I was extremely surprised at just how much help and support BSMS offers students struggling academically or socially. Drop-in centres and academic tutors are always at hand to help. And as for teaching time, lecturers are free and willing to help you via email or even meeting up – the benefit of being part of a small medical school.

What I love about medical school

There's no denying that us medics are cliquey. No surprise considering we spend most of our time together segregated from the rest of the university – the positive result of which means you get to know everyone in your year very well. Sports are a lot more enjoyable and casual rather than other militant university teams. Socials get huge turnouts and are very regular ensuring you'll always have time for some fun. This laid back approach provides a perfect equilibrium to the demanding academic side of medical school.

Every day we learn something new; we go into detail I thought didn't exist. Studying medicine keeps you on your toes. I love challenges and the one that medicine provides gives me an opportunity to reach my full potential both academically and in society. How better to learn than to actually experience what you'll be doing for the rest of your life? Thus patient contact provides an unparallel insight into what life post-medical school will be like. What's more is that patients often share their experiences of doctors and the NHS with you. It is through their past that you can develop your future, learning from others' mistakes.

As for cadaveric dissection, it has changed my entire perception of anatomy. You forget when you're at it with the scalpel that you're slicing what used to be a living human. You start to value the significance one small slipup could potentially have on a person's life.

What I hate about medical school

Medics are ridiculously competitive. Fact. Regardless of where you go you'll always be competing; whether it's for a place at medical school or a place as a junior doctor. So get used to it! But instead of viewing it as something negative, use it to your advantage. Let it fuel you to greater success. The workload you will be faced with may often seem as large as Kilimanjaro, as I have often discovered. But the only way to overcome it is to take one step at a time. Map out your work with the most important and earlier deadlines taking priority. That and time management are the simple solutions.

Some lectures may seem extremely irrelevant or even just common sense; namely those on consultation skills, basic psychology and even molecular cell biology. However, people with much more knowledge than I have formed the course so appreciating their relevance in the grand scheme of things may help you benefit from them. For example, it's a well known fact that medical students' consultation skills get worse over time as they focus their energy on the greater medical knowledge acquired and ignore patient psychology, so these lectures do prove important even though they may be as intellectually challenging as watching '*Deal or No Deal*'. And molecular cell biology, I'm sad to announce, helps us to understand the underlying causes of medical conditions, which is crucial in planning treatment. Of course there'll be some aspects of medicine that you'd prefer to avoid, but you get the luxury of choosing to avoid it once you graduate.

Some hate the fact that life as a medic revolves around other medics. Live with them, go out with them, lectures with them and the list goes on. But I've spent 18 years living with my family and I'm not bored of them so I don't really see where the issue lies.

Most valuable experience

By far the first ever conversation I had with a patient. In the oncology ward, a 68-year-old woman sharing her moving story of the role the NHS played in battling the tumour of her larynx. In a desperate financial time for the NHS with criticism always looming around the corner, this lady couldn't fault it at all. She was eternally grateful to all the staff and felt the need to name all the professionals she had been treated by. From speech therapists to consultant oncologists, she named them all. And she named more occupations in the NHS than we even knew existed ourselves.

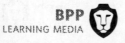

The beauty of this experience was that it showed me that one day I'd reap the fruits of my labour. It's not all doom, gloom and whining patients when you hit the clinical scene. Meeting someone who showed so much gratitude made me value the NHS so much more. Though not perfect, it saves several people's lives each and every day who otherwise would have died. And it does it all for free. Prejudice, social status and income are all thrown out of the window. Despite the fact that we always direct our attention to the flaws of the NHS, in truth most of the world dream to have that which we take for granted.

Least valuable experience

At the time, 8,000 words of reflective writing across the year didn't seem particularly valuable. However upon discovering you have to complete a similar reflective portfolio as a Foundation doctor, I began to value its purpose. I can't really say there's any experience I've had at medical school that hasn't been very valuable, and when questioning fellow students about the issue, they couldn't pinpoint one either. That just pays tribute to how well BSMS have managed to structure a relatively new Medicine course.

The future

Unfortunately the future doesn't look too bright for doctors. New government policies are aiming to increase our retirement age by one to three years and reduce our pension schemes by up to £200,000. With the way secondary care currently works, it's extremely hard to work in a hospital with normal working hours. In other words, if you plan on having a family, primary care is the way forward with the potential to work four days a week with steady working hours for a good salary. And for that reason the closer you get to finishing your degree the more attractive primary care becomes!

But as long as you're not just in it for the money, then medicine will remain as rewarding as ever. That's the beauty of pursuing a life of supposed selfless service to others. And that's what's fuelling my aspiration to practise medicine in a less economically developed country at some stage in my career – helping those who need the most and have the least.

Ten things I wish I had known before starting medical school

1. Do not underestimate how hard it is to get in. No matter how good you are: 11A* at GCSE, 3A* at A level and God's gift to academia, you'll still be in for a tough ride. It's not just how much work experience you've done; it's what you learn from it that also matters.

2. This is no time to hide under the covers. Sell yourself! You've often only got one or two shots at applying to Medicine so there's no room for the faint-hearted. Believe in yourself and in your application. Be proud of your achievements and don't be shy of making them known. But never lie on your application. Admission staff are extremely experienced, having read through thousands of applications. They'll be able to sift out lies with ease.

3. Choose your universities carefully. You'll be there for the next five to six years. Make sure you not only like what the course has to offer you but what the city does too.

4. Work hard, play hard. Don't assume because you're going to take on one of the toughest degrees around you won't have a good time at uni. These years will be the best of your life.

5. Enjoy your pre-clinical years while you can! Don't get me wrong; clinical years are brilliant but also a lot busier! So make use of the spare time you have to start off with.

6. Cadaveric dissection is essential. I cannot understand how students can learn detailed anatomy without it. Absolutely irreplaceable if you ask me.

7. You are not alone. Seek help when you need it. Universities offer comprehensive support. And if that fails, sap the wisdom and experience of the older years.

8. Be wise about attendance. If you keep in mind that lectures are compulsory then you'll be less tempted to skip many. In actual fact, the more you skip the more work you'll have to do in the long run.

9. Avoid comparing yourself with other students. This way you won't get thoroughly disappointed when you struggle. And it'll keep you rooted to the ground when you're doing well.

10. Seize the moment. Many people would give an arm and a foot to be in your position. So pursue it in a dedicated fashion. Enjoy every minute and capture every opportunity with both hands.

Practical Guidance Tips

- Every medical school has different benefits and short-comings. Focus on the good and don't let the bad get to you.

- Be the first to seize opportunities to deal with patients. These people will shape your perspective.

'Durham does have an epic Med Soc which is great at organising social events!'

Name:	Michael William Mather
Age:	22
University:	Durham University
Programme:	Five years
Year:	2
Extra info:	I am particularly interested in neurology and neurosurgery

Hello! My name is Michael and I came to Medicine after studying Natural Sciences for one year at Durham University. I am currently in my second year of Medicine and have enjoyed the last few years tremendously! I decided to contribute to this book as I hope to give you a picture of life as a medical student as I have experienced it. I cannot emphasise enough how much I have enjoyed the last few years, but my particular hope for you, the reader, is to gain a realistic insight into life as a medical student to see if this lifestyle would suit you too.

How it all started

My medical career did not start in the traditional way. I am originally from a small village in rural Northumberland and did not have any particular ambitions in my formative years but I remember being fascinated reading through various books on a huge range of subjects. I think for some time I wanted to be an Egyptologist, then an antiques dealer, then even a documentary maker. I was especially interested in nature and history.

Originally quite a slow learner in school, I eventually (after many years!) noticed I had some aptitude for maths which increased my interest in the subject. This, combined with my passion for nature, led me to take a strong interest in science. I was fortunate enough to have a particularly enthusiastic chemistry teacher who further inspired me to follow a career in science. I was encouraged to take A level chemistry while still studying for my GCSEs. I achieved 8 A*s (and 1 A) at GCSE and from here I won a scholarship to board at Rugby School; birthplace of the eponymous game. While there, I continued on track for a career in academia, studying the sciences, maths and philosophy, achieving A's throughout. Having applied for Chemistry at Oxford (and failing miserably at interview), I was matriculated to the College of St Hild and St Bede at Durham University to read Natural Sciences.

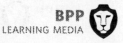

As much as I enjoyed Natural Sciences, I soon began to feel as though I was narrowing my interest too rapidly – studying microstructure of proteins did not seem terribly important when I could not even tell you where in the body the human liver is! I also began to see that a career in science would not allow me to work with people as much as I would like, so, after some deliberation and rapidly organised work experience at a GP practice in Northumberland, I decided to apply for medical school.

Application

Unfortunately, a nice and convenient course swap was out of the questions so I had to apply again through UCAS. I had to write to my old teachers at Rugby School to ask for references for my new application and quickly sort out sitting the UKCAT exam. This was all quite a hectic time but in the end I managed to get the application completed and submitted, along with several weeks of really enjoyable work experience at the GP practice.

As I had already come to know my friends from Hild Bede very well by this stage, I decided that I only really wanted to apply to Durham medical school so I could continue to live in Durham. However, still disappointed in my Oxford Chemistry interview, I decided to have another shot there as well.

The weeks drifted by as I plodded on with Natural Sciences checking my emails religiously, awaiting news from UCAS regarding a decision on my medical school application. Eventually, I was invited for an interview at Oxford. I recall having four separate interviews where I was questioned on everything from the ethics of euthanasia in the elderly to save NHS funds, to how we might investigate whether slugs have emotions.

Sadly, yet again, I must have given some rather silly answers and was rejected. Nevertheless, I was glad, financially speaking, as I had already signed a rental contract for a house in Durham by this time anyway.

Several more weeks passed when I was finally invited for interview at Durham's medical school. Durham University is in fact split across two campuses, one in Durham city and another some thirty miles south in Stockton-on-Tees (Queen's campus). Whereas most of Durham's courses are in the city itself, Medicine and some others are situated in Queen's Campus. Consequently, I travelled down to Queen's Campus for a fairly informal interview. I was quizzed by two interviewers on topics such as my motivation to study Medicine, as well as some ethical situational judgment tests. All in all, it was actually quite an informative process and I was thrilled to later receive an offer.

It is perhaps worthwhile mentioning at this stage a little bit of information regarding the medical degree at Durham. Historically, Newcastle University was actually a college of Durham ('King's College' – not to be confused with the London King's College), and this is where all medical education in the region occurred. When Newcastle became a University itself, Durham ceased to train doctors, until the formation of Queen's Campus. For over a decade now, Queen's Campus has offered a pre-clinical training (ie year 1 and 2 of the medical degree). Subsequent clinical years are undertaken under the aegis of Newcastle. Indeed, the degree one receives at the end of the 5 or 6 years is a Newcastle one – not a Durham one (despite spending the first two years with Durham).

Life as a second year medical student

My pre-clinical years were amongst the best of my life. Despite hearing stories from friends at other universities, I definitely think that Durham has to be one of the best places in the UK for a good 'student experience'. The collegiate rivalry causes immediate and profound college loyalty and it is extremely easy to get to know lots of people very quickly. Also, living in college is great because it means that you mix with people on all sorts of different degree programmes – you do not just become part of the legendary medic clique which exists at many other universities. Having said that, Durham does have an epic Med Soc which is great at organising social events!

Some students report feeling something of a division between students from Queen's Campus and those from the city, but in reality this is over emphasised and joked about. Generally, the two student populations mix very well, and if you are interested in joining lots of sports and societies, you will probably end up spending quite a lot of time in Durham city itself (as this is where most university facilities are). There is a free inter-campus shuttle bus so transport is not really an issue.

In terms of work at the medical school, Durham is quite traditional. We have fairly little patient contact, relative to the anatomy and physiology lectures we have. There is also a strong emphasis on the importance of good communication skills and the sociological theory underpinning modern medicine. Anatomy teaching is excellent, taking the form of small group tutorials around prosections (usually groups of about six). You can expect to be spending quite a few hours each week in the dissecting room (DR)!

Many other aspects of the course, such as MiC (medicine in the community) and PPD (personal and professional development) also take the form of small group tutorials which lets you have really good discussions and you definitely feel as though you can ask questions if you do not understand something.

Physiology lectures are often accompanied by practicals in the lab, which are especially good if you are interested in pursuing a career in academic medicine. We also often have clinicians come to give lectures from local hospitals (eg North Tees or James Cook hospital),

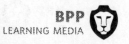

who are often very good at putting the anatomy / physiology in a clinical context, which certainly makes it much more interesting.

The timetable at Durham is really quite demanding and you should expect to be on site between 9.00am–5.00pm, with associated homework time in evenings – especially the night before anatomy sessions!

Because the year group is so small, staff get to know everyone very quickly – you can certainly expect to be chatting to many of the staff on a first name basis within your first couple of weeks. This can be especially nice if you like feeling like part of a community.

One final thing that I would recommend you thinking about early on in the degree is whether you plan on intercalating or not (that is, taking out an extra year to gain an extra degree). This can help improve your job prospects after graduation, particularly if you are interested in applying to an especially competitive specialty. It is also an opportunity to explore a subject you find interesting in greater depth – often encompassing a research project. At Durham and Newcastle intercalated degrees are optional, but it is definitely worth thinking about so you can effectively plan your undergraduate years. I believe the typical times to intercalate at Durham and Newcastle are after the second year (to get a BSc) or after the fourth year (for an MRes).

Social life

As I have alluded to previously, the collegiate lifestyle at Durham is certainly conducive to a good social life! From day one, you are introduced to so many new people that you cannot help but makes friends in Freshers' week. Additionally, the colleges, Med Soc and many other groups put on lots of social events to keep your social calendar busy. These might include nights out, college bar crawls, competitions (pub quiz style!) and days away (eg to the beach!). I could literally write a whole book on Durham's social life, but suffice to say you will definitely find something you like.

Even if you are not really a 'party person', Durham has a crazy number societies and sports clubs to keep you busy. Popular choices include rowing, cricket, football, netball, rugby, fencing, film soc, wine soc, cheese soc, skydiving soc, DUCK (Durham University Charities Kommittee), etc – the list is endless!

Expectations versus reality

I think most people come to medical school not really knowing what to expect; this was certainly the case for me. I had worries that the workload would be unbearable, I was worried about being on such a long course and accumulating lots of student loan, and also about how I would cope learning from anatomical prosections. On the other hand, I also anticipated getting really involved in all the activities the medical school has to offer, making some new friends, and generally have a great time!

It turns out that the workload is not really all that bad – so long as you plan ahead and keep on top of things, you will definitely have time to have a social life and interests outside of medicine! With regards to the student loan, sadly this is indeed one of the down-sides of medicine (but hopefully a doctor's salary when they reach consultant level is somewhat mitigating). As for the anatomical prosection teaching – it is soon something one becomes accustomed to and you will come to see what an invaluable help they are to improving your knowledge of the structure and function of the human body.

None of the medics I know regret choosing to go to medical school and most people certainly enjoy a balanced life – juggling a busy timetable with a great social life. As a rule of thumb, medics are very friendly and you will get to know people in your class very quickly.

What I love about medical school

So many things! I especially like knowing that what I am learning about will actually be useful to someone one day. Although it sounds a bit geeky, I also really enjoyed physiology in the pre-clinical years because it gives you the knowledge and understanding to make sense of things you will come across later in your clinical years.

It is also brilliant working with such a diverse range of people everyday. Although you have the constancy of your fellow students, which is nice in itself, you will meet many different patients each day who all add to your holistic learning experience. This interactive method of learning is definitely one of the best things about medical school.

To talk all about work would be an unrealistic representation of life at medical school. Everyone has a social life, and not many other degrees can compete with the social life of a medic! The friendliness and exclusivity of the medical student population means that you are always surrounded by people you know and can have a laugh with. This is probably one of the things I love most about medical school.

What I hate about medical school

I would not say that there is anything I hate about medical school. Well, except maybe the occasional 6.00am start! At times, especially when you realise you are still less than half way to graduations, it can seem a bit demoralising. However, when you

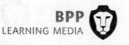

think what a good time you are having as a student, the fact that the degree is so long does not really seem to matter all that much.

Most valuable experience

The most valuable experience I have had as a medical student has been getting to know patients and my colleagues better over the last few years. There is so much to learn from everyone, and so much enjoyment (most of the time!) in getting to know people, this really is one of the most important parts of medical school, in my opinion.

Least valuable experience

There is not a 'least valuable' experience as far as I can tell – you learn something new from every situation if you think about it enough. Maybe waiting for the bus to travel between Durham and Queen's Campus seems like less valuable time; but even then, it is a good opportunity to catch up on reading!

The future

I think that despite the doom and gloom in the media about the NHS, we can still expect a bright future. People have always, and will always, need doctors – so as long as that need is there – we will always have something to do. Working as a doctor is one of the greatest privileges you can have and I cannot think of a more rewarding career. It is uniquely challenging; academically, socially, mentally, physically, and in so many other ways but most people never look back and have an excellent life in medicine.

I myself have tried to keep my options open but I am particularly interested in neurology and neurosurgery. For me, this area of medicine has made impressive advances but there is so much potential to do more. I find this prospect hugely attractive as a career specialty and hope to learn more about these fields as I progress through the degree and beyond.

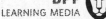

Ten things I wish I had known before starting medical school

1. Being able to drive will save you lots of time.

2. Bring a diary and calendar to medical school – you need to be organised.

3. Read some anatomy and physiology before starting the degree; it will make the first weeks seem less daunting.

4. Keep in contact with friends from home, especially non-medics! They will keep you sane.

5. Learn to cook some basic, healthy meals!

6. Devise and stick to a budget.

7. Don't buy hundreds of books, only essential core texts should be owned.

8. Come to medical school with lots of enthusiasm.

9. Talk to staff if you are having troubles, particularly early on in the degree.

10. Get involved in as many extra-curricular activities as your time permits.

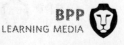

Practical Guidance Tips

Learning

- Spend as much time in the anatomy lab as possible.

- Work in the library – you are less likely to get distracted.

- Start revision early!

- Do not underestimate the importance of the more sociological aspects of medicine.

- Show an interest in what you plan to work in early (ie join Surgery Society, or MSF or community outreach schemes etc).

Living

- When cooking, make huge portions, divide them up, and freeze them so they can be quickly defrosted on days when you do not have the energy to cook.

- Car share – it saves on petrol.

- Try to catch up on sleep on weekends.

- Say hello to lots of people on campus. Knowing lots of people helps you feel at home.

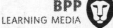

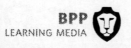

Chapter 3

The third year: A dose of reality from five medical students

Syed Muhammad Tahir Nasser

Emma Gees

Penelope Cresswell

LE Dawson

Leyla Swafe

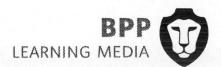

The third year: A dose of reality from five medical students

'Whenever people ask me what degree I'm doing and I reply 'Medicine', they always wince. Then they ask, 'So how many years left?' 'Three' I say, smiling wryly and nodding as if to say "Hey, someone's gotta do it, right?"'

Name: Syed Muhammad Tahir Nasser
Age: 22
University: University College London
Course: Five years
Year: 3
Extra info: I find Medicine fascinating

I was never your typical medical school applicant. I had not wanted to study Medicine since I was teething. I did not imagine walking around with a stethoscope, taking blood and smelling of antiseptic soap. I still do not know what the profession of medicine will be like, though the blurry picture has become a tad sharper.

Am I going to go through every step of my medical school application in this narrative? No. I am however going to give you the highlighter-version, the dime-tour. Having had to apply twice through UCAS, having taken seven medical school interviews, six of which were Oxbridge, and having gone through the Bloody Miserable Admissions Test (aka BMAT) twice, I have gained at least a small insight into the hell that is medical school admissions. Rest assured, any pain that you've gone through / are going through, people have experienced the same – and come out the other side…

How it all started

'Why medicine?' is a weird question because looking back, the only reason I can pick out as to why I chose Biology and Chemistry A levels over other subjects was because Medicine was the hardest course to get into, the most notoriously gruelling and ultimately the greatest challenge. I therefore accepted the challenge, and wanted to keep open the door to that possibility.

Eventually it came down to a simple decision – English Literature as a degree or Medicine. Those were my two options. To say that my parents had no role to play in my decision to choose Medicine over English Literature would be a lie – of course they did. Looking back,

 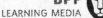

I'm immensely glad that I did choose that path as I have realised that what I loved about English Literature was not quite the study of stories – but the writing of stories myself. That is a hobby I still avidly pursue and so I've managed to keep the best of both worlds.

I have said why I didn't choose English Literature, but not why I chose Medicine. Honestly, I don't know. I did two years of work experience in a care home and a week of clinical work experience and still had no idea what to expect in medicine (any medical school applicant who tells you that they know what medicine will be like is either deluded or lying). Aside from that, you don't need to be mad over the idea of medicine before you even consider it. There will no doubt be other people in this book telling you that you need to be crazy about medicine before you go into it. For some people that was possible – for me, it just wasn't. I liked the idea and I was interested and determined enough to pursue it as a degree even into a second year of application, but I could not say more than that.

That all changed when I got into medical school. The first lecture on the course was about the extracellular matrix that fills in the gaps between the organs of the body and holds it all together. Stupidly basic and I was thrilled to be learning about it. I was dumbfounded by the idea that I'd simply never questioned exactly what the cement of the body was. I'm lucky in that within the first lecture of my medical training, I knew I was in the right place.

Application

Perhaps it was the lack of obsessive enthusiasm that failed to impress the university admissions in my first year; I failed to get any offers and was forced to take a gap year during which I re-applied. I applied to Oxbridge both years along with predominantly London universities followed by one or two outside London. I applied to them because, by the grace of God, I had done well in exams and felt that I had a shot at getting into some of the top medical schools. The total rejection I faced from all six university applications was quite shocking – up until then, I'd never so miserably failed at anything! I took it quite well – in fact, I practically shrugged it off. As the rejection letters started coming through the post, I was increasingly thinking about taking a gap year. The day before the last rejection letter came, I raised the issue of a gap year with my parents who weren't too keen on the idea. When the last rejection letter arrived, I laughed and told them I'd got my way!

I should perhaps make a mention of the UKCAT and BMAT at this point. Sitting in a booth at a 'Kaplan' test centre while trying to figure out which geometrical shape is comparable to another geometrical shape, while the voice in the back of my head was asking '*what on Earth has any of this got to do with medicine?*' was quite frankly, exasperating. With further

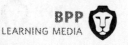

preparation, I managed to get a score of 20 or 21 or so on the BMAT the following year and suddenly received interviews from every single medical school I applied to; a good medical admissions test-score can work wonders.

Life as a third year medical student

At present, I am on the Orthopaedics (fractures) and Rheumatology (Lupus) rotation and as such have to be in hospital (which is luckily a minute's walk away) for 8.00am trauma meetings. These are meetings in which everyone received through A&E the previous night are gone through with all the doctors / registrars / junior doctors and medical students present. After that, each doctor gets a different patient and they all go off to meet their patients in a ward round. This is where the stereotypical medical student runs around on the heels of the consultant and gets ceremonially grilled.

'Clerking' patients is the bread and butter of all medicine and surgery and is often the most daunting task for a new clinical student. It consists of approaching the patient, obtaining consent, taking a medical history of both their recent reason for coming to hospital and past medical history, before conducting the relevant clinical examinations. Clerking is a skill that you will only really master after many, many years of practising medicine. It is a skill that requires the doctor to process information while writing it, think about the next relevant questions in light of the information already gathered, extrapolate differential diagnoses and investigations required to ascertain a diagnosis – all while also talking to the patient in a directed yet conversational manner!

In terms of teaching time, I get approximately five hours of lectures a week (one hour a day) and perhaps one or two tutorials a week on a particular condition relevant to that rotation. Aside from going into hospital, I will do about one and a half hours of private study a day (it's the beginning of the year at the moment – it will go up to about three hours a day at some point). In terms of free time, you get as much or as little free time as you want as it's up to you to work hard. We have a mock exam in January which doesn't count for anything and then exams at the end of the year that count for 60% of our quartile ranking at the end of our medical degree (say what?!). The exam consists of hundreds of single best answer style questions and a practical exam called an Objective Structured Clinical Examination (OSCE) where they bring in actors who pretend to be ill to test your clinical skills under time pressure.

Social life

This is entirely subjective depending upon the individual. Personally, I despise nightclubs. I won't rant about why because I have a limited word count. As such, my 'night outs' consist of going with friends to a restaurant, going to a comedy club to watch some stand-up or just going and getting some ice cream. As this is to be juggled with going back home and meeting family, one gets to go 'out' about once a week, at best. To be honest, going 'out' is entirely up and down – some weeks you go out more and some weeks you don't go out at all. It should be noted that I still do plenty of extra-curricular activities such as participating in university clubs and societies and attending events; while medicine does indeed limit your social life, it shouldn't disable it. There is no such thing as a 'normal' life so don't wonder '*Am I going out enough*?' If you are happy with your social life, that's all that matters.

Expectations versus reality

As stated above, I never really had an 'expectation' as to what it would be like. Prior to doing medicine, you don't really have any frame of reference so having an expectation is rather difficult. I didn't expect that I would be so involved in university clubs and societies as I am now, but that is something that I have chosen for myself.

I didn't expect medicine to be such a big topic. Sounds stupid, I know, but prior to going into medicine, it is almost impossible to imagine the breadth and depth of topics involved. That may sound daunting but it should be something that excites you to a certain degree as one comes to realise that there is something for absolutely everyone in medicine.

An additional factor that I didn't expect was how many people come to medical school. The result of this is that you develop many acquaintances but only a few truly close friends, as one is continuously thrown into different working groups. The ability to work within a team of people whom you don't know very well becomes crucial even at the early stage of medical school.

What I love about medical school

Medicine is really my first answer. Don't get me wrong – I don't like having to cram my brain with hundreds of lists – but the content can be really really fascinating at times. More than that, medicine is highly relevant. It is always applicable to the world around us and to the people around us. Knowledge which is only relevant but not fascinating is always tedious; knowledge which is irrelevant but interesting is intrinsically worthwhile but ultimately meaningless and finally knowledge which is both relevant and interesting is that which jumps off the page.

In an egotistic sense, medicine is also a very highly sought-after profession. Mothers from India to China to the Americas hope that their young daughters marry a nice, handsome 'doctor' (change inflexion as

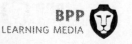

appropriate to accent) and women too, entering and competing in the once male-dominated profession are viewed with respect and a degree of admiration. In fact, I have a friend (I'm not going to name him) who gets a certain kick every time he tells someone that he is studying medicine! One should be careful though; applying to medicine for the prestige is not going to cut it. Medicine is long and gruelling and if the only thing that is keeping you going is your ego, you're inevitably going to give in at some point.

What I hate about medical school

The dog-eat-dog nature of the beast. Perhaps this is just my medical school, but we are provided with no past papers for help towards the exam. As such, a river of black market past papers is handed from the older years to younger years. Admittedly, by the time the revision period comes around, everyone has access to the papers through word of mouth, but often individuals get left behind and suffer the consequences.

The length of time that a medical degree takes is also rather annoying. Whenever people ask me what degree I'm doing and I reply '*Medicine*', they always wince. Then they ask, '*So how many years left?*' '*Three*' I say, smiling wryly and nodding as if to say '*Hey, someone's gotta do it, right?*' There is however, a reason that the medical degree is so long – there is a lot to learn!

Medical students often complain about the competition and that can be annoying, but the fact of the matter is that each student only got into medical school by being competitive; competition is an inevitability and is invariably useful as it drives up the standard of knowledge. This competitiveness can however, on occasion, give birth to a paranoia which manifests itself as 'herd mentality'. Individuals who know that they could do better through, say, independent study, instead of attending every single lecture, will nevertheless attend every lecture – bored off their faces and not benefitting from it at all – simply out of the fear of breaking away from the 'pack'.

Most valuable experience

Doing an Intercalated BSc in Physiology was undoubtedly my most valuable experience. It enabled me to understand medical research from the point of view of a scientist as opposed to a medic and that is an important distinction. The distinction lies in that the medic is often only interested in the disease insofar as it affects the patient while the scientist is interested in the mechanisms of physiology and disease, often entirely independently of the patient! Both have their own advantages and disadvantages.

The value of a BSc is multi-faceted. From a strategic point of view, it gets you an extra degree which may not be of great benefit on the MTAS form, but will be on your CV for jobs down the line. Additionally, the BSc acts as a gateway to the scientific research profession. An increasing number of medical doctors are developing research careers simultaneously, so as to provide their patients with the most scientifically up-to-date treatments. A scientific BSc in which laboratory work is undertaken also gives one the opportunity to work at the frontier of scientific developments. It teaches essential skills, such as the ability to read a high volume of research papers quickly, while extracting the key 'take home messages'. Moreover, the dissertation at the end of the year hones the skills of writing scientifically – an ability that differs greatly from other forms of writing, requiring a greater attention to detail while yet maintaining a logical thread.

Least valuable experience

Honestly? Oh boy… this could get me in trouble… pre-clinical-medicine lectures. Let me explain what I mean by that: at UCL, the medical degree is divided into a pre-clinical (first two years) and clinical (last three years) with a BSc slotted in the middle (third year of six). The pre-clinical side is devoted entirely to the study of medicine from the perspective of the textbook – that's good to a large extent. It gives a thorough grounding in the basics of medicine from a scientific perspective. Unfortunately, it is all taught in a lecture format whereby one lecturer stands and speaks in front of 300-odd students. I just don't learn from a lecture. The only thing it achieves is to make me sleepy and tires me out so that I can't do any substantial work once I get home in the evening.

The future

My thoughts on the future have invariably changed over the past three of four years. I am now studying in the hospital and seeing future versions of myself in the form of foundation year doctors who run around performing jobs for registrars and consultants. That is now a prospect looming on the (still fairly distant) horizon.

I have not, thank God, had any frustrations or disappointments regarding my choice of medicine. Invariably in life, there will be a few, and the trick is (in my humble opinion) not to make a career in medicine the defining feature of one's life. It is important to value things outside of one's career and this is perhaps neglected by medical students more than all others, as medicine is like a monster – it has the habit of eating up everything else in one's life. The trick is to strive for a good work-life balance. At certain points in one's career, this balance may inevitably be tipped temporarily one way or the other. At that time, it is useful to have an understanding

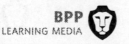

partner who realises that the reason you're too tired to talk to them when you get home is not because you don't love them, but simply because you're too tired.

In hindsight, so far I can say that I made the right choice with medicine and I have no regrets in having chosen it. Where do I see myself in ten years? No idea; I do not have enough experience to choose medicine or surgery at this point. I might possibly be a specialist registrar working my way towards a consultancy post or possibly, with the way the world is going, I may find myself in a post-apocalyptic nuclear wasteland, infusing myself with drugs to counteract irradiation sickness. Only time will tell.

Ten things I wish I had known before starting medical school

1. Work hard for the BMAT / UKCAT / GAMSAT.

2. Get the past papers for every exam.

3. Research from the year above which textbooks to get and use them.

4. Use USMLE question databases to practise medical questions.

5. Some of your friends will be earning £40K as investment bankers while you are about £40K in debt.

6. Five years will go quicker than you think.

7. Don't try and fit in with everyone else – you will lose your own personality in the crowd!

8. Keep up extra-curricular activities as far as possible – they will keep you sane.

9. In the interview, don't say you want to become a doctor because you want to help people.

10. Don't become a doctor if you don't want to help people.

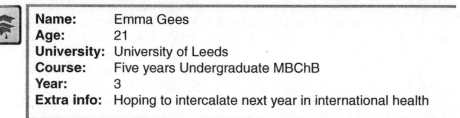

'You are no ordinary student... you are a medical student'

Name:	Emma Gees
Age:	21
University:	University of Leeds
Course:	Five years Undergraduate MBChB
Year:	3
Extra info:	Hoping to intercalate next year in international health

I'm Emma and I'm a third year at Leeds. I came straight to university from school (no gap yah for me) as a fresh faced 18-years-old with no idea what the next few years of medical school had in store! I have non-medical parents, who go weak at the knees at the thought of blood!

Outside of medicine I love sports including squash, running and ballet. I also write for the Leeds Medical Magazine.

I wanted to write for this book as I think deciding what you want to do in life is one of the most difficult decisions you have to make and I wanted people to know what it's really like to be a medic. I love writing as well so the idea of writing about my experiences of medical school really appealed to me!

How it all started

As a young child I decided that I wanted to be a nurse and insisted on constantly wearing a nurse's outfit (my mum had to buy multiple copies). When my sister was an infant she used to have febrile convulsions and so spending time in hospitals further fuelled my interest. (I felt sorry for the poor doctors who used to let me play with their stethoscopes). As I grew older, like most prepubescent girls I become obsessed with animals and so a vet became the career of choice. My grandparents own a farm and although I loved animals I realised that sticking a hand up a cow's backside at 3.00am and being outside in the depths of winter really didn't appeal.

At 15, my school sent everyone off on a week of work experience and I found myself at a local hospital. I was hooked from the word go and I realised that this could be quite a 'cool' career to pursue. I liked how there was always something going on and how it gave you potential to make a difference in the world. I love talking and people so the idea of spending everyday interacting with other people and meeting individuals from all walks of life appealed enormously. I also liked the detective side of medicine, working out why people have certain symptoms (or maybe that's because I've watched too much 'House'...). Finally,

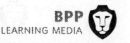

medicine seemed like a secure career that would allow me to travel and would mean I would always be needed, regardless of where I am.

Before I started at medical school, I spent a few weeks out in Uganda and I was shocked by the contrast to UK hospitals. However clichéd, it reaffirmed that medicine was what I wanted to do in life and showed how much needed to be done to help everyone have equal access to basic healthcare. It also deglamourised medicine and showed the blood, sweat and tears that go into life as a doctor.

I wasn't sure what to expect of life as a medical student, just that it would be hard. When I mentioned my career aspirations to people I tended to get raised eyebrows and a knowing look, as if they knew what I was letting myself in for. I asked my grandfather (a retired orthopaedic surgeon) what he thought of my plans and chuckling he said: 'Well, it's a rather barbaric career really isn't it?'

Application

I can be really indecisive, so the fact my choice was limited to 29 universities was a blessing in disguise. I then crossed off universities which were more than a few hours from home (wanted to avoid expensive train tickets home), which left half a dozen or so to pick from. Visiting the universities helped to try to get a feel for the place, however I hadn't liked Leeds when I visited and only put it down as my family said it had a 'good' reputation and it wasn't too far from home.

No matter what anyone says, applying for university is stressful and the word UCAS fills your stomach with butterflies. I felt as if someone sitting at a desk somewhere was playing with my future. As non-medical applicants starting receiving offers I became a bundle of nerves, worrying what I had done wrong and what I would do next time. Medical schools have hundreds upon hundreds of applications to look through so it can take a fairly long time before you hear back, so don't worry! As I used to think: 'no news is good news'.

On interview day at Leeds you could smell the panic in the room full of students, all of whom were desperate to impress and to secure an offer. However, everyone seemed friendly, which calmed my nerves. Before I knew it my name was being called and as I stood up to respond, the fire alarm shrieked through the entire building. Like a sheep I followed the flock of students down the stairs to the ground floor, where we all huddled out in the cold – waiting for the noise to stop. During my return trip to the aptly named 'Room X' I managed to get lost on one of the many staircases that seem to spiral up to nowhere. On my arrival, looking rather red faced, I was greeted by my interviewer who was clearly not impressed by my distinct lack of orientation skills. Matters were made

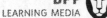

worse by my entrance into the interview room when I promptly tripped over the threshold and went flying into the student interviewer, who was rather good looking. Thankfully, the rest of the interview went well and I was delighted when I received an offer from Leeds. It goes to show that interviews don't go as badly as you think and are there to 'get to know you' more (and to check you're not the next Harold Shipman).

Before interviews make sure you have looked at the type of questions they could ask and think about how you can respond to a question you don't know. Just be yourself and be honest – the interviewers can spot dishonesty from a mile off.

Life as a third year medical student

As one of the sub-deans said on our first day: '*You are no ordinary student... you are a medical student*'. This may sound like something from an M&S advert but his words do have some truth to them. Our course can be challenging and fascinating in equal measure, meaning it can sometimes be difficult to leave behind at the end of the day. While all other students often have fewer hours than they can count on two hands, medics are 'blessed' with a packed timetable that is just as bad as a schedule from school.

One of the most common things I heard in Freshers' year was '*Oh well, you only need 40%... this year doesn't count*!' Unfortunately for medics it does count (and you usually need higher than 55% too I'm afraid).

In the third year we start placements full time (Mon–Thurs), with self-directed learning and lectures on a Friday. We have four rotations (elderly, GP, surgery and medicine) of five weeks plus lecture weeks in between. On a usual day I'm awoken from my blissful slumber at 6.30am. It's still dark outside and non-medics are still fast asleep in bed. Most of them probably rolled into bed a couple of hours ago and may have no intention of waking before noon. After a quick cup of coffee it's a race to catch the shuttle to the hospital, for an 8.30am start. Placement can finish from anytime from 3.00pm to 6.00pm depending upon what's going on. Placements are scattered across the whole of west Yorkshire, from Leeds, to Halifax to Bradford. The medical school provides accommodation for placements further away and is available at all the hospitals outside Leeds (except Harrogate where a daily coach is available). There is also £50 to cover transport costs for the year.

From day one we are expected to show professionalism in every aspect of our degree. We are future doctors and there is an onus on us to conduct ourselves like that. This responsibility is further highlighted when we start clinical placements in the third year as we are now 'student doctors'.

We are expected to dress and behave in a manner that fits our future occupation.

Despite all the hassle (and the long days / early starts!), placements can be such fascinating and enjoyable experiences. We get to see patients and learn clinical skills which will be used throughout our career. Who wants to be stuck in a lecture theatre when you can be watching surgery in an operating theatre? Placements are a reminder to medics that there is a light at the end of the biochemistry tunnel. This is what we came here for and this is where it all starts... someone pass me my stethoscope please! The work load in the third year is fairly large, however if you stay organised it shouldn't be a problem. One of the changes from the second year is the reduction in lectures (less than one per week currently!). The onus is now on us to do self-directed learning, finding out about conditions and treatments in our own time around placement. There are several SSC projects due in throughout the year: ethics, a pre-Christmas one and one in the summer after exams. They provide a chance to do something slightly different to the usual subjects, including learning a language, learning tai chi and spending two weeks with the police. Exams wise, we had a spot test in October and then the OSCE and the integrated exam at the end of May. I have heard that the OSCE and integrated are generally fair exams and as long as you practice on the wards you should be fine. I felt the spot test allowed us to demonstrate our knowledge but because everyone did so well, the pass mark was over 60%. Anywhere else in the university, this would be a 2:1!

Social life

I go out around once a week because I find it hard to 'go out' and then turn up to placement as if I'm tired I can't function! However, I know people who still do go out on a very regular basis. I'd much prefer to go to a pub with friends or go for dinner than go out clubbing so we tend to do that. We try to meet up on a very regular basis, which is nice after a long day at placement.

I don't think I have a less active social life than people on other courses, but I think I go clubbing less. I found it difficult in the first year as all my flatmates went out every night and would return home at 4.00 or 5.00am. I tried to go out with them as much as possible in the first couple of weeks and soon realised that 9 o'clock starts and very frequent late night sessions weren't a perfect match. So, I started socialising more with medics as we had the same timetable and so went out on nights suited to our more hectic days.

Time management is key to fitting in work and play; you don't want to be the one not going to the MedSoc night as you've not finished your essay due the next day. But, by being organised you can have your cake and eat it!

I'm a bit of a 'keen bean' and do lots of extra-curricular stuff. This year I realised I was doing too much and had to say 'no' to several things. Societies are a great way to meet other people, especially non-medics and provide relaxation time away from the world of medicine. Don't get me wrong, I love the course but at the end of the day I like to switch off and ballet and squash allow me to do that.

Expectations versus reality

I arrived at medical school with little idea about what it would hold. One thing I was worried about was the workload and was concerned that there would be little time for other things. However, I soon realised that the workload is manageable, particularly if you don't leave it all to the last minute. In the first few years there is a large amount of contact time and you can be in from 9.00am to 5.00pm. This is frustrating as other people seem to have days off at an end, but it gets you used to the long days, that you will have once you get on placement.

At school we were used to being top of the year and felt like big fish in a garden pond. Arriving at med school was like a tadpole being thrown into the sea. Everyone seemed really clever and I found the content we covered difficult to grasp. We are used to getting A's in everything and at university the bar is raised. The pass mark is 55% and a C (a grade that would have seemed like the end of the world at school), now becomes the expected standard. This can be hard to get used to, but once you realise that a C is good and is what is expected, people start to relax.

What I love about medical school

One of things I most love about medical school is the people I've met. Almost everyone on the course is friendly and I have made some great friends from the course. Medics have a reputation for being cliquey and I can see why people say that, but I think we're close because we're all going through the same things together. I also like how many opportunities are available to us – there are so many things within the medical school going on, from research to charity work (bike rides, pub crawls, volunteering) to sports and music groups.

Leeds has a range of students from all walks of life: from mums and dads, to former nurses, to 18-year-olds to 'career changers' in their early thirties. I really like it as it means everyone has different experiences and brings something different to the course.

What I hate about medical school

One of the things I found most difficult when I arrived at Leeds was the lack of support. I had come from a school where we all had supportive form tutors who helped us through the trials and tribulations of UCAS and A levels. At university, we arrived and none of the lecturers / facilitators knew our names or anything about us. If something had gone wrong I wouldn't know who to turn to within the medical school. However, Leeds has recognised this and has recently introduced a tutor system where we meet regularly with a personal tutor and they have provided advice about where to turn if things aren't going well. This is important as medicine can be a demanding degree and can take a lot out of you. We are also regularly confronted by issues of life and death on placement. Medics are one of the professions most likely to have mental illness including depression and substance abuse!

Something else that I dislike about medical school is the competitiveness. To get into medicine you have to have some level of competitiveness and I think the course provokes it more. When we apply for FY1 jobs in the fifth year, we are ranked according to academic ability and so from early in medical school some people seem determined to do better than others. It is important to remember that a grade C in med school (around 60%) is the same as getting an A outside of medicine.

Most valuable experience

Doing badly in an exam is not what most people would consider (at first glance) to be a valuable experience. However, after the highs of Freshers' term, it brought home the reality of life at medical school. We are used to sailing through exams at school and scraping a pass made me realise what level of work would be required. It was a hard exam and I wasn't the only one who did badly: around 40% of the year failed the exam. I think this was because we hadn't acknowledged how much work and preparation is needed before exams. As the lecturer pointed out, what we learn now will be applied to our clinical practice later on. If we knew less than 60%, would we really be in a position to treat patients?

The experience taught me not to take things too seriously and that if I did badly, it was pain but it wasn't the end of the world. If I did fail, it would mean I didn't know enough to treat a patient, which would be unfair on them. Re-sitting would provide the opportunity to reconsolidate my knowledge and ensure I know enough to treat patients.

Least valuable experience

The idea behind 'Personal and Professional development' (PPD) is to check we're not all robotic doctors, with no feelings for our patients.

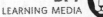

However, the vast majority of people at medical school aren't robots and so don't gain much from the sessions. It is important to reflect upon our experiences, but the way we are expected to, is so artificial that it makes the exercise pointless. Furthermore, we need to submit a reflective log at the end of the year that is assessed. How can someone mark someone else's thoughts and feelings? People end up writing utter rubbish or writing what they know the marker wants. This defeats the whole object of the exercise.

The future

Three years into medicine, I am thoroughly enjoying the course, with its challenges and rewards. I have a long way to go, but the finish line seems closer. Medicine is such a fascinating course, where we have the chance to make a difference. However, it is such a long course and stamina is required! At the end of this year, most of my non-medic friends will be graduating and starting jobs and moving on with their lives. It's strange to think they'll be joining the real world while I'm still in student limbo for another couple of years.

Finance is a difficult issue and I can't wait until I receive my first pay cheque as a FY1. I'm already fed up of being dependent upon other people and being in so much debt. I feel fortunate that I only had to pay the lower tuition fee level. I don't see how people can afford to do medicine with the recent increase it tuition fees. The rise will push those from lower socioeconomic groups out of the picture and discourage graduates from applying, since they have already had to pay for one degree. Medicine is a profession where you will encounter individuals from all walks of life and if individuals from poorer / less typical backgrounds were pushed out of medicine, then the medical profession would not be a true reflection on society. I hope the government realises this before it is too late.

Before I came to medical school I was determined to be a psychiatrist. Now, although I find it fascinating, I don't see myself spending my life in that career. I like the idea of being a GP, where you develop a relationship with your patients over years and can see a wide variety of conditions. You need to be a 'jack of all trades'. I also hope to work abroad in the developing world, maybe with MSF (Médecins Sans Frontières). I speak French so hopefully that will come in useful.

I don't think I have any regrets about medicine. I can moan at times, but in reality I love medicine and the highs compensate for the lows. If you think medicine is for you, go for it. The application process is a nuisance and can be very stressful but, it is worth it!

Ten things I wish I had known before starting medical school

1. Everyone is in the same boat, worried that they're not good enough to be here, so don't worry about it!

2. Medicine is one of the hardest, but most rewarding things I've ever done.

3. Be prepared to work hard, but party even harder.

4. Medicine is expensive: the textbooks, the placement clothes, the travel expenses...

5. Don't be scared of consultants who try to put you down. Ignore them and rise above it.

6. Third year rotations are great fun, but also very exhausting and take up so much time!

7. Don't be put off by the application process, you will get there one way or another.

8. If you don't know an answer, be honest. Trying to bluff will just cause you more embarrassment.

9. If you are struggling with anything, talk to someone. Don't suffer in silence!

10. Don't buy all the books on the book list, look at them first in the library before deciding which ones to purchase.

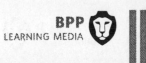

Practical Guidance Tips

How to pick medical schools to apply to:

- Look at grade and subject requirements (no point wasting a choice if you don't meet the requirements).

- Play to your strengths, if you've done well in UKCAT apply to universities which take it more into consideration or vice versa.

- Look at the course type: do you want traditional, PBL or integrated?

- London or not London? London is very expensive and if you're living on a budget it might be easier to go to university away from the capital.

- Look at the area; do you want to be close to home or six hours away on a train?

- Look at size of the medical school: do you want to be in a class of 330 or a class of 130?

- Do you want to be in a big city or on a campus in the middle of the countryside?

Five things to do before leaving medical school:

1. Travel, especially if you didn't have a gap year. Make the most of the long holidays in the earlier years (they get shorter later on).

2. Explore the area around your med school, you'd be surprised what there is to do.

3. Get involved with societies.

4. Take up a new hobby.

5. Do something for charity – there are so many things you could do with your University's RAG: sponsored walk, do a charity bike ride, climb Kilimanjaro, volunteer with a local children's group... the list is endless!

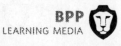

> *'I've had some ups and downs, but for me, it is all I can imagine myself doing.'*

Name: Penelope Cresswell
Age: 20
University: Cardiff University
Course: Undergraduate Medicine MBBCh 5-year course
Year: 3
Extra info: I aspire to specialise in care of the elderly

I came into medicine straight from school. Worried about getting a place, and not wanting to spend a year of my life away from education, I was keen to apply and get started on my career! Now a third year medic at Cardiff, I am loving the course. But I am also just starting to appreciate how tough the next few years are going to be. I have had some ups and downs, but for me, it is all I can imagine myself doing.

How it all started

There is something exciting and unique about medicine which I have never been able to find with anything else.

I can't really pinpoint when my interest in medicine began. There is no background of medicine in my family, and I was never really exposed to hospitals as I child. All I remember from visiting the doctors as a child is the toys in the toybox! And yet from a very young age I knew it was what I wanted.

Maybe it's because I have always loved learning. Thinking back to primary school I loved how everyone wanted to learn. I have such fond memories of sitting in the classroom with no one laughing at you for asking a question, or sneering at you when you did well in a test. Secondary school was such a big change. Suddenly there was that hierarchy in the classroom – do well and you were a 'geek'. I really hoped that coming to medical school would be a new start. I hoped it would be a place for learning where we all want to study and achieve, with no one getting put down for wanting to do well.

And I have always had big expectations of myself. I am lucky in the respect that I have always done well academically, and it's true I wanted to choose a career which made the most of my strengths. But it had to be the underlying spark and passion I have towards medicine that lead to me being a medical student today.

Application

Applying to medical schools was a ridiculously frustrating and stressful time. The application process is tough. Some people hear back really quickly. Others have to wait a long time.

It had been four months when I finally heard anything from a university I had applied to. Apart from a postcard from Cardiff which read '*Please be patient...*' it had been silent. My life started to revolve around me checking my emails!

Something I never thought about before I applied is other people applying to university. We apply earlier, we often hear back later. Also, despite having the good grades you are not guaranteed offers. It can be pretty tough when everyone asks you what university you are going to and all you have is silence or rejections, especially when everyone is expecting you to do well.

I was rejected by all four universities I applied to. I had two interviews – one at St Andrews (which went disastrously!) and one at Cardiff. The Cardiff interview was incredibly friendly, and more like an informal chat – a complete contrast to the formal St Andrews interview!

Southampton and Peninsula rejected me straight off (though all waited until March to let me know – giving me a tense six months of waiting).

I was later thrown a lifeline by being placed on the waiting lists of Southampton and Cardiff. This meant a lot of anxiety and uncertainty, and a rather difficult and disappointing results day despite getting the grades I wanted. Frantic results day phoning of the waiting list numbers gave no joy. Then, a week before Freshers started, Cardiff phoned me up and offered me a place.

Looking back at the application process it is not something I would like to repeat, but it is just the first step in a series of trials you will face in medicine. It is always going to be competitive.

I think that my experiences have made me appreciate my place at medical school even more. I have fought to get here, and it has given me a great determination to succeed and prove that it was the right decision to make me a Cardiff medic.

Life as a third year medical student

The third year is an exciting time. Apart from a few days in the first year, and a couple of weeks at the end of the second year, this is my first clinical experience. After two years of almost solid lectures to get out seeing patients and medicine in practice is more than welcome!

Don't get me wrong – we still have lectures, near-on 200 in fact. That is a lot to learn alongside spending time on the wards, not to mention reading around the subject.

The way it works is we have three blocks of placement – each eight weeks long. Each one is a different specialty and can be in any south-east Wales hospital – but with the free buses they kindly put on for us up to the third year it really isn't too bad!

A typical day from my surgical placement:
06.45am – Get up and get ready
07.10am – Leave my house
07.30am – Catch the bus
08.00am – Join ward round
10.00am – General ward work
12.00pm – Lunch
13.00pm – Consultant bedside teaching
14.30pm – General ward work
17.15pm – Catch bus back
18.00pm – Get home

There is no getting away from the fact that it is a high workload. But that comes as a given with medicine! Trying to fit an hour or two of work in a night is the ideal. However, after getting home from placement you are shattered – and quite often before you even open your textbook your head has hit the pillow!

Before we start placement they bring us back at the end of August (that's right – no more long summers) for three weeks of lectures and introductory talks, and we have more lecture weeks scattered throughout the year. When placement is on, Wednesday mornings are dedicated to four hours of lectures and tutorials. The afternoons are dedicated to sport etc (a luxury we do not get from the fourth year onwards).

A particularly interesting part of our curriculum is the Oncology project (a six-month project from October to March where we follow a patient with cancer). This follows on from our Family Case Studies in the second year where we followed a family, and gives a great insight into patients' experiences of medicine.

As for our favourite topic – assessments! For the third year we have two written papers around April time, along with the first of our practical exams – the OSCEs. We also have a data interpretation exam (interpreting X-rays, ECGs etc) in February and medical evidence coursework (critically appraising research papers etc).

At the moment these seem pretty daunting, particularly OSCEs as they are the unknown! And sometimes it seems like every consultant tells us something different! They are fair exams though as long as you prepare well for them.

It's worth noting that it can be a shock at first when you go from getting 90% at A levels to 65% at medical school, and go from being top of your class to average. That is just the competitive nature of medicine, and if it happens to you don't worry! If you get into medical school, it means you are a very intelligent person competing with other very intelligent people. There is no shame in not coming top!

Social life

Your social life is what you make of it. Despite misconceptions, you do have some free time (especially in the first two years) but you need to use that time wisely! I struggled the first two years to find the right balance! In the first year I didn't go out as much as I could have done (I got this major guilt complex that I should be working and not going out!), and then in the second year I went a bit too much the other way!

Something which I discovered early on is that we do have time to go out, but at different times to all other courses. It can be very frustrating when everyone else is going out but you have coursework or exams to prepare. Then finally when you have some free time everyone else seems to have exams going on. This can put quite a strain on your friendships with non-medics and can become very frustrating when living with non-medics.

Extra-curricular involvement is important, but for me I have always found it quite hard to get involved. I am one of the least sporty people (quite atypical in my cohort!) and so sports were out of the question for me! There are loads of societies you can join, but many aren't built to fit around a medic timetable. It does limit your options, and make it more difficult for you to commit to something, but find a passion and you can stick with it.

Expectations versus reality

The one thing I have really been disappointed with about medical school is that you lose the closeness and relationship that you had at school with your teachers. Agreed being a class of 300 compared to a class of 30, there is no way that the academic staff can know everyone, but it was quite a transition to suddenly feel that you are just one of many.

And I wasn't expecting the extreme toll that medicine was going to have on me. I knew that medical school would be hard, but I have to say I wasn't quite expecting it. The exams are tough – rightly so, but have led to me breaking down in tears. At times it is mentally and physically exhausting.

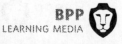

I have had to go above and beyond what I ever thought was possible. It has taken time to adjust but I now feel more ready for what lies ahead. I think it is a process that every medical student has to go through.

What I love about medical school

There are so many things I love about medical school. One of the biggest things is the friendships that I have formed. It is an intense course and we all need to go through it together. It is great to be spending time with like-minded people and to learn from each other. You really feel part of a family in Cardiff. Despite the year group being large there is a great feeling of continuity between us and you really feel like you are part of something.

As far as the course goes, patient contact has to be one of the best parts. We are very lucky to be in a position to get so much contact with patients, and even as students we can make a difference to their experience. It is great going out on the wards, talking to the patients and having the time to listen to them. You hear some very interesting stories on the wards!

And I absolutely love what I learn. Every so often when you are going through your notes you find an interesting fact that ties everything together. Medicine is a puzzle, and it really excites me that the puzzle pieces are beginning to fall into place. I look back at myself as a first year to now and I can't believe how much I have learnt.

What I hate about medical school

Sometimes I wish I could be another student for a day. Our course is intense and our timetable is packed. It is a big undertaking and some days, especially living with non-medics, you can't help but start to envy them for their free time and more relaxed lifestyle.

Talking of envy though, it can work the other way. I hate the fact that being a medical student can lead to people automatically making assumptions about you. True, in anything you do people form an opinion of you before really knowing you. But the reputation that some medics have of being arrogant and keeping themselves in the medic 'clique' can mean that it can sometimes be hard to make friends outside of medicine.

The short holidays are never easy. I live about five hours away from Cardiff, and so popping back home every weekend is simply not an option. This makes the holidays even more valuable to me and so it's getting increasingly tough as the years progress. And unlike other courses, we don't get much study leave at all. This year I have ten days. This means you can't rely on the study leave and if you are a crammer then try and get rid of that habit now!

Most valuable experience

Surprisingly, my standout moment in medicine so far was my week on nursing placement – a week dedicated to us looking after the patients under the watchful eyes of nurses. It gives us the time to spend with patients that as medical students and as doctors we just won't have.

It was such an amazing insight into life as a nurse and gave me a huge appreciation for what they do. There is always this big stigma about doctors looking down on nurses, and in fact some students have apparently seen this week as a 'waste of time'. But understanding the other professions we work with so closely is so important to us.

I guess another reason I enjoyed it so much was because it was my first proper clinical exposure. It was the first opportunity I had to follow patients' progress over a couple of days and get a real feeling for clinical practice.

Least valuable experience

At medical school, time is at a premium. We are so busy that any free time is golden and has to be used wisely. So when we are on placement and clinic is cancelled there is suddenly a dilemma on our hands. My least valuable experience has to be wasting time on placement. It is incredibly difficult to be doing something all the time. Some hospitals are great and schedule many teaching and learning experiences for you, others not so much. But when a clinic is cancelled, and you turn up on the ward to see the lonely F1 trying to cover all the patients on their own, suddenly being 'pro active' is very difficult. We try other wards but they are full of other students. We take histories but most we have taken already, or the patient has refused. Suddenly you find yourself at a bit of a loose end.

The one thing I have really learnt from this is that it is ok to go to the library and not feel guilty about leaving the wards. Ward experience is invaluable and that is where we learn the best, but when there is no one to teach us then we inevitably have to make the best use of our time and sometimes that means book work.

The future

Despite everything, I absolutely love being a medical student, and I truly believe I will love my career in medicine. I aspire to specialise in Care of the Elderly, as this is an ever important specialty which covers such a broad area of medicine.

One major worry is when I will find time to have a family. It is not going to be easy, but I am determined to make my career and family plans work together. I may down the line take a year or two out for this, but otherwise I can't see myself taking any time off. I think I would be quite bored without medicine!

I do sometimes regret not doing another course at university – having the chance to study but also have more time to experience life outside university. But those regrets are soon diminished every time I go on placement. I definitely made the right choice choosing medicine, and I cannot wait for my future career as a doctor.

Ten things I wish I had known before starting medical school

1. It really is a lifestyle not just a course – your identity becomes that of a medic, not a student.

2. Doubts keep creeping up on you – don't ignore your worries but keep in mind that everyone has them.

3. A levels are easy in comparison – it really is a big step up. A really, really big step up!

4. The course is at times very emotionally draining – expect to have low times and remember that it is nothing to be ashamed of.

5. Make sure you make non-medic friends at the beginning!

6. It is not just a five-year course. It is a commitment to at least the next ten years of your life in training, and you may have to put the rest of your life on hold in the meantime.

7. Fellow students can become very competitive. Be careful who you share your ideas with.

8. Despite moaning about early mornings, complaining about long days – we wouldn't have it any other way! In fact, I reckon I'd be so bored doing a course with only a few lectures a week.

9. Don't go crazy and buy every single textbook! I spent a good few hundred pounds of my shiny new student loan in first year and regretted it ever since!

10. Medic socials involve a lot of fancy dress – so remember to bring the face paints and make sure you get as involved as you can – because medical school is above all else great fun!

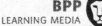

Practical Guidance Tips

- Don't let medical school overwhelm you. Take it slowly and remember hundreds have been there before you and made it!

- Get out and join societies in the first few years. You may want to test the waters with the workload first, but remember that there is time to have a life outside of medical school – you just need to get the balance right!

> *'Keep focussed, stay organised and you'll be fine!'*

Name:	LE Dawson
Age:	24
University:	University of York
Course:	Five-year MBBS
Year:	3
Extra info:	Pharmacology BSc (Hons) University of Newcastle upon Tyne

I am what one might call a post-graduate student. I guess that implies that I am old and mature. Well, I hope to dispel this rumour and give you a fair and reasoned piece on why I entered medicine; what trials, tribulations, and ultimately joys have occurred in the early stages of my medical education. I have decided to share my experiences to highlight that there is no stereotypical medical student and that no one should be deterred from applying, unless you really don't like ill people.

How it all started

My background is pretty straightforward: I went to a state school and enjoyed all subjects I studied, and was arguably a bit too keen, leaving me unsure which A levels to choose. I am not from a medical family, my father is an airline pilot and my mother trained as a midwife; my mother claims that my great-grandfather was a successful doctor, but I've not seen any proof. In essence, I don't really know where my inspiration to become a doctor came from. Perhaps it was my unhealthy obsession with the TV show '*Grey's Anatomy*' and wanting to find my own '*McDreamy*' or, perhaps just ultimately biology was my favourite subject. Anyway, it was safe to say that medicine seemed a viable career choice. As A levels approached, however, I realised that I really didn't enjoy chemistry and consequently presumed medicine would be impossible. After much deliberation I decided to pursue a Pharmacology degree; avoiding REDOX (*reduction-oxidation*) calculations but still maintaining some clinical science. In the summer prior to starting my first degree at Newcastle, I started a job at a local hospital as a healthcare assistant. This gave me a wealth of experience in healthcare, from daily ward duties, to day-surgery and minor injuries, I saw it all. Observing medical professionals made me realise that actually medicine was for me. I decided to continue my degree and develop some further work experience; after all, knowledge of pharmacology would probably come in handy one day!

Application

Fast forward three years and I was ready to graduate and start the UCAS application and interview process... again. The disadvantage of being a post-grad applicant is that you have to sort out the UCAS process independently without the input and careful guidance from a school support structure. I doubt the process has changed too much over the last few years, but the biggest hurdle was writing the personal statement, or rather condensing it down to 4,000 characters. Deciding where to study was slightly problematic and consideration about the financial implications were noted. I did contemplate graduate courses; as there is funding available throughout the four years. I was deterred from this route due to the competitiveness and the intensity of the course; Medicine seemed challenging enough without the need to cram five years of work into four. In the end, I applied to one graduate entry course and three normal undergraduate courses. Everyone has different criteria, but my decisions were mainly based on geographical location and the popularity of the course, so I chose schools that had a favourable applicant to place ratio. I didn't really give much thought to the traditional versus problem-based learning (PBL) styles as I thought that the same work would be covered regardless, but many of my peers have strong opinions on this matter.

I was subsequently offered a place at the Hull-York Medical School (HYMS) which, I have to admit, was bottom of my four choices, mainly because there was the danger of having to study in Hull. After I accepted this offer, I found out I was indeed going to spend a large majority of my time at Hull!

HYMS is one of the newer schools that received its first intake in 2003. As I'm sure the prospectus will tell you and as the name implies, HYMS is split across two university sites. This means that for the first two years you are predominately based at either Hull or York following exactly the same curriculum and with lectures video-linked between the two lecture theatres; on the whole this works remarkably well with only a few minor technical glitches. You are grouped into small PBL, clinical skills and placement groups with the aim of working together to achieve weekly 'outcomes'. This style of independent learning took a while to get used to and I wasn't particularly a fan at first as the process of learning seemed unnecessarily prolonged, and could easily be shortened by spoon-feeding us the same information. I have, however, come to realise what a valuable skill independent learning is. Personally, it has encouraged me to ask more questions and engage with clinicians to obtain information. One of the highlights of the week in Years 1 and 2 was clinical placement, in which we were introduced to history-taking and clinical examination in primary and secondary care. This early exposure is unique to HYMS and really does prepare you for the commencement of clinical years.

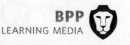

Life as a third year medical student

....No lectures?!

In the third and fourth years, students are required to rotate between other hospitals in the region: Hull, York, Grimsby, Scunthorpe and Scarborough every six months. We study in blocks of eight weeks attached to a teaching firm; each block is dedicated to learning a particular system. Each week focuses on a particular topic, for example: 'child with a fever', which builds on previous knowledge to cover common causes of paediatric febrile illness, identifying signs, symptoms, appropriate investigations and management plans. We are also required to clerk relevant patients and present them to seniors. Resultantly, an average week in the third year varies, but generally consists of the following aspects: an early ward round where we would often be questioned on X-rays and ECGs. Here it is a sensible idea to begin looking around the bedside: general demeanour of patient, any clues to diagnosis (nebulisers, oxygen, vomit bowl), medication and basic observations that are recorded, this helps develop a comprehensive assessment of the patient. We are expected to regularly attend clinics with our lead consultant. Most of this time is spent observing, but it is interesting to see how out-patients are managed in secondary care. Afternoons are often spent in ward or classroom based teaching. Here we are shown some interesting clinical signs and symptoms to stimulate our reading, and discuss management and problems encountered that may affect us as junior doctors. At HYMS, we have a large exposure to primary care which, typically, equates to a day a week. Here we see general clinics and are required to take histories and examine a variety of patients with common GP ailments. The rest of the time we are required to clerk patients, spend time in acute admissions and complete our outcomes. By Friday, it is time for the infamous 'academic discussion forum': an hour-long telephone conference between the other hospital sites in the region. This is intended as an opportunity to speak to other students with interesting cases and iron out any problems encountered during the week; however the session is often littered with long, awkward pauses as students avoid questions from the lead tutor. Our timetable is very much 9.00am to 5.00pm, Monday to Friday and permits 'self-directed learning' which means we can, to a certain extent, develop our own ways of achieving outcomes, whether on the wards practicing skills, in the library (or at the gym). I would advocate some out-of-hours work in the hospital; this is where some of the most interesting medicine happens. In the evenings, about two hours is spent reading up on pathologies encountered during the day. However, as the sun sets, so does my concentration and the television is turned on.

Assessment consists of a series of formative exams throughout the year and completion of an OSLER (Objective Structured Long Examination

Record (clinical assessment)) every eight weeks on the current block, with the serious summative exams at the end of the third year. As a PBL-led course, there are very few lectures in clinical years, but every three weeks we have an afternoon in university covering the topics of pharmacology, prescribing, and therapeutics. Additionally we undertake three-week intense student selected components (SSCs) throughout the year, ranging from clinical specialities, to more art-based subjects like photography to broaden our horizons as future clinicians.

Social life

Work hard, play harder

The well known phrase 'work hard, play hard', is frequently spoken about medical students. This is pretty accurate. It is important to get a good work-life balance and is imperative to pursue interests outside of medicine to divert from the intensity and stress that this sort of course entails and also makes you more adept at connecting with patients as a human being. First and second years were probably more lively and involved going out at least twice a week. This dwindled as clinical years progressed, attendance at 9.00am ward rounds were required, and the guilt of appropriate professionalism kicked in. I spent the lower years developing extra-curricular interests and got involved with the sports teams. Every medical school has a multitude of societies to get involved in, so it's all individual choice. HYMS is a relatively small medical school, so you really develop friendships with students and staff alike, something perhaps lost at bigger medical schools.

Additionally by rotating placement every six months, I got to visit many parts of Yorkshire and Humberside I would never otherwise have the chance or opportunity to experience (who knew Grimsby had a sandy beach and Pleasure Island is minutes away?).

Expectations versus reality

Patient perspective

My biggest preconception was about Hull. This was fuelled by the statistic that Hull is one of the most deprived places in the UK. Indeed, it does have large areas of deprivation, as most large urban areas do but, from a medical point of view, the variety of medical conditions presenting in this city is extraordinary and it is really intriguing how patients and their co-morbidities vary throughout the region. I can safely say that from a student perspective, Hull is lively, cheap and there are always friendly faces to be found. York offers a more refined cultural experience, but this all comes at a price!

What I love about medical school

The medical profession is very exciting to be a part of; healthcare is forever changing with continued research and innovation, which will ultimately have a massive impact on society. There are not many people who can claim to be part of this, so there is an element of prestige that I am proud I will one day be part of. I also love the social side of medicine: though everyone has different backgrounds we generally abide by the same ethos and appreciate when to have a good time, while developing the strong camaraderie that is needed in stressful environments.

What I hate about medical school

One of the problems studying medicine is the constant feeling that I should be working or worrying that others are working more than me. This is to be expected as medics are constantly faced with assessment and examination. It is important just to realise that everyone works differently and to ignore the scare-mongers amongst the year, particularly during exams. The requirement to move every six months is also rather tiresome and it does feel like I'm living out of a suitcase half the time. However, treat this as an opportunity to meet new people and learn about different towns. The hospitals in the region all vary, so while it takes time to get used to the new trust protocols, naturally competency is improving and is beneficial for the future. However, by far my biggest grievance about studying medicine is the fact that my friends are all earning and I'm still not! While some are buying houses, cars and going on exotic holidays, I spend my holidays figuring out a revision timetable and dreaming of my first pay-packet.

Most valuable experience

There are many valuable experiences that you pick up on while progressing through medical school. One of the most valuable things I have learnt is that I had a tendency to avoid areas of medicine that I disliked or found challenging. Cardiology was an area that intimidated me and I felt very poorly equipped to tackle this subject. I decided that the best way to overcome this fear was to immerse myself in cardiology during an SSC. It was daunting and at first I knew absolutely nothing which made me feel inadequate to the point of doubting my ability as a future doctor, but this intense immersion in the subject meant things soon started falling into place. I learnt that problems avoided are not problems solved and an element of self-doubt can be advantageous; as to question and review ones actions may lead to better patient care in the long run.

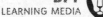 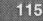

Least valuable experience

The least valuable experience is probably in relation to the horrific amount of non-clinically related forms we have to submit: self-appraisals, peer appraisals, tutor appraisals, critically appraised topics, quality improvement projects, reflective essays... the list goes on! They are all immensely boring and not the sort of medicine I expected. However, becoming a good reflective doctor seems to be on the agenda for the future and will occur in interviews.

The future

Initially, I was so preoccupied with actually getting in to medical school that little thought was spared for my medical future. It did start to worry me when asked if I was an aspiring medic, surgeon or general practitioner and my default answer was always 'it's too early to tell'. This answer seemed suitable in first year, but as a third year I was concerned I had yet to find my niche, particularly as it was becoming apparent that many of my peers had career paths in mind. I used the SSCs as an opportunity to develop interests outside of the core curriculum, focusing on subjects such as accident and emergency, radiology and anaesthetics. I've recently developed a keen interest in paediatrics, and enjoy the added challenge of interacting and building rapport with anxious children and parents and being able to legitimately avoid using medical jargon. Of course, it is also much more fun examining Teddy first! I am still predominantly concentrating on my short-term future and focused on passing finals so I can enjoy an elective abroad. I should probably be worrying about Foundation Schools and pensions, but that's for the newspapers to bemoan. Ultimately, I know that medicine is more than a job, it's a way of life and despite the endless work, early mornings and fear of causing harm I have absolutely no regrets in having chosen this path. I know that one day I will be able to travel anywhere in the world as a doctor, so all the blood, sweat and tears will all be worth it and I look forward to successfully treating my first patient!

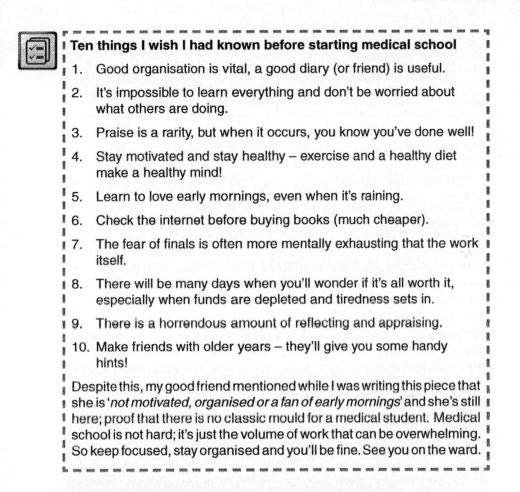

Ten things I wish I had known before starting medical school

1. Good organisation is vital, a good diary (or friend) is useful.

2. It's impossible to learn everything and don't be worried about what others are doing.

3. Praise is a rarity, but when it occurs, you know you've done well!

4. Stay motivated and stay healthy – exercise and a healthy diet make a healthy mind!

5. Learn to love early mornings, even when it's raining.

6. Check the internet before buying books (much cheaper).

7. The fear of finals is often more mentally exhausting that the work itself.

8. There will be many days when you'll wonder if it's all worth it, especially when funds are depleted and tiredness sets in.

9. There is a horrendous amount of reflecting and appraising.

10. Make friends with older years – they'll give you some handy hints!

Despite this, my good friend mentioned while I was writing this piece that she is '*not motivated, organised or a fan of early mornings*' and she's still here; proof that there is no classic mould for a medical student. Medical school is not hard; it's just the volume of work that can be overwhelming. So keep focused, stay organised and you'll be fine. See you on the ward.

Practical Guidance Tips

- Make friends with the older years, they will give you invaluable advice about exams, clinical contacts and revision aids. (Oh, and remember to offer them a drink as finals commence).

- Do not be intimidated by the volume of work or others around you. Just get on with it and do your best. No one will fault you for that.

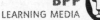

'Hearing and reading about the demands of medical school, I certainly knew that Medicine would not be a stroll in the park; in fact I was prepared for five years of hard work and little play.'

Name: Leyla Swafe
Age: 23
University: University of Aberdeen
Course: Five years
Year: 3
Extra info: Originally from Sweden

My name is Leyla Swafe and I am 23 years old. I am currently in my third year of Medicine at the University of Aberdeen in Scotland and I am expected to graduate in June 2012. Having lived in Sweden for almost all my life I thought it would be an exciting experience to study abroad which is why I applied for Medicine in the UK.

Choosing to go into medicine (or any other degree for that matter) is a big decision as you will be spending at least five years in medical school. When I first decided to go into medicine I was not sure what to expect. The student profiles on the university web pages always appear to be sugarcoated, I therefore thought this would be a great opportunity to give an honest and personal account of what it is actually like to be a medical student at my university.

How it all started

In school, I really enjoyed social sciences, but as time passed my interest declined as I quickly realised that there were people who were far more suited to potentially becoming world leaders. At about the same time I re-discovered an interest in science subjects, particularly biology. The human body was the most interesting topic in biology, so naturally the thought of doing medicine was implanted in my mind. From an early age I have enjoyed studying and acquiring new knowledge and since medicine is a lifelong learning process, it made it even more of an attractive option. I also spent six months in the Accident and Emergency department working as an auxiliary nurse, which added to my interest in medicine, and as unoriginal as it may sound I did find it very rewarding to put patients at ease.

I was told by family friends who were doctors, to become a dentist instead as it involved less work and potentially more money. Nevertheless, I could not stand the thought of studying the oral cavity for the rest of my life when I could be studying the entire human body. Lastly, the

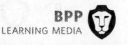

fact that Medicine virtually guarantees you a job also influenced my decision and today it is a relief knowing that I will probably not, unlike many of my friends who are not studying medicine, be struggling to find a job. Hearing and reading about the demands of medical school, I certainly knew that medicine would not be a stroll in the park; in fact I was prepared for five years of hard work and little play.

Leaving your home country for five years is certainly a challenge and at times it has actually been a lot more difficult than I expected it to be. When I first arrived I experienced a bit of a cultural shock. At times it has been difficult to integrate with the British students and even after four years I still find it easier to be with people in my own situation, which is probably why most of my friends are non-British students. I also find it frustrating not being able to see my friends and family whenever I want. Many of my classmates live only hours away from Aberdeen and can easily go home over a weekend. Sure there are times where I feel that I regret choosing the UK to do my degree, but then again, being taken out of your comfort zone can be a valuable experience in many ways. At least I am happy about the medical school, and at the end of the day I am thankful my university accepted me into Medicine.

Application

As I did not have biology as a higher level subject (International Baccalaureate) the UK universities I was eligible to apply for were limited. I applied to UCL and King's because I wanted to study in London, and Manchester because I liked the prospectus with the opportunity to study a foreign language alongside medicine. My fourth option was Aberdeen because it was in Scotland which meant I did not have to pay tuition fees as I was from an EU country.

I was desperately waiting for a letter to come through my letterbox giving me an interview date and checked my UCAS application every day dreading a rejection. My first interview was for Manchester University. Unfortunately I made the mistake of not preparing enough and my recollection of the interview was a rather dreadful one. My interview date for Aberdeen came rather late (April) and by then I had already had three rejections (didn't get an interview for the London universities). Needless to say, there was a lot of pressure on me to perform well this time. I did spend more time preparing for this interview which I believe paid off. Answers to standard questions were well rehearsed and I probably sounded quite silly answering the 'why medicine?' with my perfect (if I may say so myself) well rehearsed reply.

Overall, I am impressed by the selection process for medicine in the UK. Although interviews can be very intimidating, it is a great opportunity for you to demonstrate your dedication to wanting to do medicine.

Life as a third year medical student

Every year of medical school is a tough one, and it really does not get easier until after finals (in Aberdeen the final exams are in the fourth year). Senior medical students would normally say that the three first years are a stroll in the park compared to the fourth year as they mostly consist of lectures and minimal exposure to patients on the wards. Most days we have back-to-back lectures starting at 9.00am and finishing at 3.00 or 4.00pm with a one-hour lunch break. However, twice a week we spend a few hours at the hospital clerking and examining patients under the supervision of a consultant. Luckily, we get every Wednesday afternoon off, whereby we are encouraged to do some sort of sport activity.

In first year I did not spend many weekends studying. Freshers, including medical students, do find the time to go out even during week days. It was a long time ago now, but I can remember being sleep deprived for most of the first year and many of my classmates, including myself, could easily nod off during a lecture. Which is fine really, however by the time exams start the stress can sometimes be overwhelming. Nowadays, when the amount of material that needs to be covered in the exams has increased compared to in previous years I at least *try* to study for a couple of hours every week.

In the three first years we also have the 'Community Course' where we have tutorials on non-clinical aspects of medicine. For four weeks we also get to do a Student Selected Component where we (in groups) get to research a topic from a list of choices that interest us. Unlike in a few other universities in the UK, it is not compulsory to do an intercalated degree in Aberdeen, however there is an option to do so in order to gain a BSc (Hons).

The vast majority of our assessments take place at the end of the academic year rather than each term. In Aberdeen we have a communications course where we are trained to communicate with patients efficiently with role play exercises. During exam time we have (apart from written exams) so called OSCEs where our clinical skills are being assessed with the help of actor patients.

The difficulty with exams in medicine is not necessarily the contents, but the quantity that you are expected to know. Unless you revise on a regular basis it is easy to forget the most basic facts. That is especially true for the clinical years where you do not want to come unprepared to a clinic, as not knowing the answer to basic questions can be very embarrassing (been there, done that).

Social life

During my time at university I have been able to squeeze in a few activities. I am a member of the dance society at my university and attend two classes per week. Apart from that I have been the treasurer for the Nordic society and I have spent some time volunteering for the Teddy Bear Hospital project. To avoid having any student debt by the time I graduate, I also work part-time at the university library. As I am also interested in research I spend a few hours a week working as a project assistant for the Epidemiology research group at my university. Needless to say, it is possible to have activities outside of medicine. I think most people who are accepted to medicine have to be fairly good at managing their time as they have probably had a few activities alongside getting the top grades that are required in order to get into medical school in the first place.

Expectations versus reality

Medicine is undeniably more demanding compared to many other degrees, and not only because of the nature of the subject. Many of my friends who are doing other degrees only have a few lectures to attend every week. However in Medicine you are required to attend lectures / clinics / wards from 9.00am to 4.00pm most days. Apart from that one *should* also be spending some time studying and revising at home. Just because lectures have finished, it really does not mean you can go home and watch TV for the rest of the day. You are always expected to do a little bit of reading every day if you want to keep on top of things (easier said than done though). However, it does not necessarily mean that medicine has to take up *all* your time. Medicine *does* limit the amount of free time you have, but if you know how to use it wisely, you can indeed fit in a few extra curricular activities. It is not only desirable for you in order to keep sane, but also encouraged for your CV.

What I love about medical school

One of the things that I love about medicine is that you rarely get bored as medicine is anything but a monotonous degree. (That is, once you start your clinical years and get to spend most of your time in the hospital (I am not a big fan of lectures)). Unlike many other departments the medical school is very well organised, almost to the point where we are being spoon-fed during the first few years of our degree (which of course involves commitment and a lot of studying on our part). In Aberdeen we have the privilege of getting a flavour of most specialties during our fourth year. We get to sit in with the doctors in clinics, go to theatre and sometimes even scrub in. In Aberdeen we are also given opportunities to work at a hospital or GP setting outside of Aberdeen *and* we get the chance go on placements in other places such as Inverness, Orkney Islands and Shetlands. For

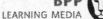

those who are interested there are also plenty of opportunities for medical students to be involved in research projects at the hospital. To conclude, Medicine can be as fun or as boring as you want it to be!

What I hate about medical school

As a medical student, I have learnt to appreciate the value of time. Therefore anything that wastes my time will inevitably annoy me. During the first three years of my degree which mainly consisted of lectures I was struggling to stay concentrated beyond the first five minutes. I rarely succeeded. Spending most of the time day dreaming, I do think much of the time I spent attending lecturers was a waste of time (unless I subconsciously absorbed the information which I seriously doubt). I suppose it is understandable that it is the most cost-efficient way to deliver information and I know that for some people who learn by hearing it does work. Personally I think problem-based learning (PBL) would be far more suitable for me, which I did not really put too much thought into when I applied to universities.

Time becomes even more valuable as the years go by and the dreadful finals are approaching and you wish you could be spending most of your time in the library instead of wasting it going to the hospital only to find out that a clinic has been cancelled. Though going to theatre is an exciting experience at first, it can be either a hit or a miss. Some surgeons would be happy to let you assist during a surgery and give you some teaching during the operation. However, you may also have to spend at least four hours standing in a corner because the surgeon cannot be bothered talking to you during a routine procedure. This is just something you will have to accept as a medical student – some days you will have learnt and seen a lot, other days you wish you had not left your bed in the first place.

Most valuable experience

I recently spent a week in the labour ward at the maternity hospital and I was given an opportunity to shadow a midwife for 12 hours. As some of my classmates never got the chance to see a delivery because their patient did not deliver their baby by the time their 12-hour shift ended, I was pleased when I, only after four hours into my shift, got to be present at the birth of a baby boy. Since it was a complicated birth, I unfortunately did not get to deliver the baby myself (which you would otherwise be allowed to do). Nevertheless it got me thinking about how lucky I was to get the chance to take part in such an important moment for the baby's parents. Being a medical student is a privilege in many ways. We get the invaluable opportunity to see and speak to people from all spectrums of life, from babies who have recently been born, psychiatric patients who tell us their personal stories, to the elderly approaching the final stages of their life. As one of my friends said, entering medical school shapes you as a person

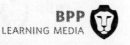

in many ways. You become more empathic and understanding, and with time and training you learn how to communicate with patients effectively.

Least valuable experience

As a medical student I have learnt how to cherish the free time I have. Once finals start approaching, weekends will not be a 'chance to relax' from a hectic week, but two valuable days where I would ultimately want to catch up on everything I have learnt so far. In one way or another, medicine is always at the back of my head which can be very frustrating at times. Unfortunately (or fortunately, depending on how you look at it) since we only have exams once a year, the stress just keeps building up until exam times. In medicine I feel as if there is a constant pressure to keep up to date with all the information I am being overwhelmed with. Not only because I have exams approaching, but also because I am going to need that knowledge to treat patients in the future. I try not letting the stress absorb me entirely by having a time-out every now and again. Taking a weekend off, seeing friends or going to the cinema does help, however I must admit that I sometimes feel slightly guilty about it afterwards.

The future

I look forward to the future working as a doctor and finally being able to use the knowledge and skills which I have spent five years acquiring (though I will probably spend most of my time doing paper work in the first year). However my optimism may well change after having worked as a doctor for a week. Foundation doctors keep reminding us to cherish our time at university, as life will change drastically once we start working, and not necessarily for the better. At the moment I am not too concerned about future pay – I was never really in it for the money – as long as I get paid enough to get by and live decently. I am more worried about the hours that junior doctors are expected to work; long shifts and nights shifts are awaiting and limits will be pushed.

Having seen many specialties already, I have a better picture of what I do not want to specialise in rather than what I do want to specialise in. I wish I could say that I hope to work within a specialty where I will never get bored, however that is quite unlikely seeing as once you are a consultant you will probably be doing the same thing in and out until you retire. I am hoping to be able to do more with my degree other than being confined to whatever specialty I decide to do for the rest of my life. Perhaps I will decide to put a greater emphasis on my interest in research and combine the two. I may become disillusioned in a few years' time; however at the moment I do feel that the sky is the limit.

Ten things I wish I had known before starting medical school

1. Having an interest in the human body and diseases is almost a pre-requisite for wanting to do Medicine. There will be a huge amount of information needing to be absorbed in a limited amount of time, and if you do not find it interesting, you will be making your life so much harder.

2. If you are in it for the money and the prestige, there are plenty of other things you could be doing, because being a doctor will not make you a millionaire and it is certainly not a glamorous job.

3. The competition is not over just because you got into medical school, it will still be in your interest to get good grades and improve your CV.

4. The life of a medical student is not always exciting. Many times you may well be ignored even if you have made an effort to come into the hospital at 8.00am and even if surgery may sound exciting, as a medical student there will be times where you will just be holding a retractor for eight hours without being spoken to.

5. Your social life may not be as good compared to other students and that is perhaps one of the sacrifices that come with choosing medicine as a career.

6. Stay active and creative. You can have a life outside of medicine and though work may seem overwhelming at times, every effort should be made to try to actively do something different.

7. Cramming in medicine is probably the worst thing you can do to yourself. If you want to avoid ageing prematurely, try to keep on top of the work.

8. Befriend senior medical students, they've been there and done that and can be of great help when you are in need of good advice (and past papers) in times of exam panic and despair.

9. Though having friends who are medics can be great for revision, it is equally important to have friends who are non-medics, discussing answers to exam questions is the last thing you want to do after an exam.

10. Enjoy your summer holidays to the maximum. Once you start working there will be no such thing as taking three months off work. If you're lucky you may get three consecutive weeks off.

Practical Guidance Tips

- If your interest in medicine stems from watching too much *'Scrubs'*, then you may want to get a dose of reality. Speak to people in the field of medicine and try to get involved in health care activities of some sort.

- Medicine is a very competitive degree. If you do not get in the first time and you are sure you want to do medicine, do not give up. Take a gap year and in the meantime and do something that can boost your personal statement.

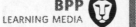

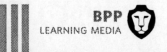

Chapter 4

The fourth year: A dose of reality from five medical students

Stephen Barratt

Neil Chanchlani

Thomas Kwan

Kristina Lee

Ross Kenny

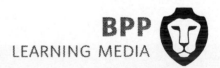

The fourth year: A dose of reality from five medical students

'As a nurse I didn't like being told what to do by the doctors. So I've committed to six years training to be a doctor – only then I'll be told what to do by the nurses!'

Name: Stephen Barratt
Age: 31
University: University of Sheffield
Course: Five-year MBChB
Year: 4
Extra info: Intercalated in my third year at Sheffield. I started medical school at the ripe old age of 25; nine months after completing a degree in adult nursing from Sheffield Hallam University. First in my family to attend university

I live three miles away from where my dear mother pushed me out just over 31 years ago (in just under two hours: '*You've always been good like that, Stephen*', my mother often tells me). I was born at the Northern General Hospital in Sheffield in 1980, the middle child to a somewhat dysfunctional family – an abusive father, a loving but highly strung mother, an older brother with 'problems' and a salt-of-the-earth, railway engineer younger brother. As a fourth year student, it seems a fitting time to look back and reflect on why I ever decided to be a medical student. I say medical student because it has only recently dawned on me that I will *actually* be a doctor. This scares me so much I have taken the day off revising cardiology for my forthcoming exams to write a contribution to this wonderful book. I hope you enjoy my story!

How it all started

From a young age I didn't want to be like my parents. My parents were both working class, as were their parents and their parents before them. Had Thatcher not butchered the industry I would have gone down a mine at 16 or been off to the Army like my dad. But with the mines closing there was a vacuum, I look back now and see it as an opportunity to be something different – and to have a choice. And this is why I wanted to be different to my parents – I wanted a choice of what to do and what to be.

Second, I wanted money. I remember my mum and dad having fierce, often physically violent, arguments about money; or the lack thereof when I was a child. We owned our own house but I had a

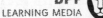

free school dinner. I went on the school trips but didn't buy a load of stuff from the gift shop. We had lovely full-length curtains hanging in the front room window but they weren't fully lined. I suspect this story resonates with thousands of families in the current economic situation. So I wanted a choice and I wanted money. So, why medicine?

I was bright at school but coming to terms with being gay and being bullied at my mining village comprehensive took more of my time than Biology GCSE. I left school at 16 with ok but not spectacular grades and won a place at Sheffield University to do a nursing diploma. I got on with girls, liked caring for people and I was at university. Happy? No. I was bored. So I left the diploma after eighteen months and I took a job in a call centre with disastrous results so I started a degree in adult nursing with Sheffield Hallam in 2002. I was coming top of my class and was very starry eyed about the doctors on the wards I was training in. They seemed to know everything and I was really impressed. I wanted to be like that: to take charge, lead the team and stop being told what to do by these doctors – and become one myself! Medicine would be amazing; I had no doubt.

Application

I applied for medicine in 2004 when the tuition fees were about to increase to the lofty heights of £3k a year. So I needed to secure my place on deferred entry so I could take advantage of the reduced fees. This was essential because I would be funding my own degree out of my student loan. Despite being on course for a very high first class honours degree, I didn't have any A levels so I never got past the first tick boxes on the application for the ubiquitous Chemistry A, Biology A, Maths A and *other* A grade A levels with the majority of admissions tutors I emailed.

I wrote a personal letter to the then sub-dean for admissions for Sheffield, Mr Andrew Raftery. I had a whirlwind exchange with him in this office and he promised me an interview and suggested '*You shouldn't mess it up!*' Two weeks later I had been interviewed and accepted to Medicine. I was ecstatic. I told my friends at nursing school and everything changed. I'm not sure if it was like being a wounded animal in the pack or whether they thought I had betrayed them by 'going over to the dark side'. This was very sad and I completed my nursing degree over the next eighteen months rather lonely and pretty unhappy.

If I may digress briefly and discuss applying to medical school: this tick box approach to applications is expected but also incredibly unfair. I interview prospective medical students for Sheffield and the vast majority are incredibly smart and impressive young people. The applicants I turn away, however, show no personality, no commitment to caring or have a clue how to show some insight, some empathy or human traits essential

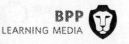

for a career at the bedside. Then again, I couldn't at 17 years old. Are we asking too much of what are, pardon the patronising, just children? Also, how can you develop the much-lauded 'people skills' when achieving these stellar A level grades, which takes so much time buried in textbooks?

Life as a fourth year medical student

I get up at about 6.00am during the week. Following a shower I eat cereal while checking *Wikipedia* for the diseases and procedures I'll see that day. When I was on Orthopaedics I would need to arrive at the hospital for 8.30am. This would entail driving 25 miles up the motorway with other students at Doncaster Hospital, getting the shuttle bus to the hospital itself, going to the medical education office, signing in and dropping my bag off in my locker. I would attend the trauma meeting chaired by a consultant orthopaedic surgeon where I might be grilled on dynamic hip screws or managing septic joints. I would then scrub in for the theatre session, holding the retractor that the registrar was too senior (superior) to hold and generally having a very enjoyable and informative time. Lunch would be a quick sandwich while attending lunchtime teaching on anything from examining the knee to rehabilitating a person with a fractured neck of femur. Then I would be in clinic during the afternoon. I would be asked to examine the new patients, present them to the consultant, come up with a management plan and then await feedback on how I performed. Clinic would end about 5.00pm and I would complete the 90-minute commute back to Sheffield. Once home, I would chill out for an hour, eat dinner and then do some more reading on the things I had got wrong today and on the subjects coming up tomorrow.

At the end of each placement we have a sign-off form about our attendance, professional behaviours and our overall clinical skills. We rate ourselves and the consultant also provides a rating. In addition some placements ask for more; Critical Care for example. You had to insert five cannulas, manage five airways, draw up five lots of drugs for injection, set up five IV infusions and so on. Furthermore, in Cardiology you had to examine a patient with a senior doctor observing who would rate your performance and complete a form stating your competence. This was repeated in Rheumatology and Renal Medicine. In GP we also had to audit 50 patients and the care they received for a specific condition.

I believe we are assessed on a range of relevant and specific competencies at Sheffield. You do feel like you're jumping through hoops and, dare I say it, ticking boxes again, but I do feel that I have gained in skill this year. The assessments keep you on your toes and make sure the medical school can pick things up if you fall by the wayside.

Social life

Being seven years older than most other people at medical school I'm not one for being out clubbing until 5.00am every night. I did all that the first time round at university and find my current social life is composed of coffee with friends, meals out and the odd trip to the pub after lectures. What curtails my social life is my income, not my course. Although having to attend a ward round at 7.30am with a pit-bull of a consultant is not something to be attempted after a lengthy session down the pub the night before! I socialise about three times a week. With a partner at home I'm conscious that I can't spend 35 hours a week on placement, 10 hours commuting, 10 hours studying and expect my relationship to accommodate me going out partying for a few hours on top of that too! I have medic friends with children who have a similar view. Something has to give somewhere.

Expectations versus reality

I didn't expect to learn as much as I have done. I also didn't realise the breadth of knowledge required and the range of practical skills you need to develop. I never thought I would be challenged to the extent I have been and that I would mature in the ways I have. Also, when I was training to be a nurse I was told that doctors are narrow-minded, cold 'medical model' orientated machines that care only for the bone, organ or wound they happened to be treating at that time. I never realised medicine was such a human vocation and how deeply caring you need to be. Dare I say more caring than a nurse? I never expected to have this view when I was a nurse myself.

What I love about medical school

I love things from the embarrassingly shallow to the deep and philosophical. Shallow in that I love walking down a corridor of waiting patients in clinic, my stethoscope sprung round my neck like a mayoral chain, watching as they think '*There goes a doctor*'. (Perhaps they just think '*Who is this clown and why does this clinic always run late*?') Philosophical when I held the hand of a 45-year-old man only days from death two weeks ago and pondered the meaning of it all and the injustice that such a young man was losing his battle with cancer. You spend so much time and energy worrying about making the grades, getting that cannula in or taking blood first time, getting the questions right, putting that suture in when really just sitting quietly and holding someone's hand in their final hours is the best doctor you can be for a patient when the end inevitably comes.

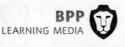

I love the variety of always learning something new. I enjoy the vocational aspects of the course in so far as learning how to do something, or knowing something, so you can then go out and make someone's life better. Coming up with the correct diagnosis is a real thrill and learning how to provide leadership to a team of people is very satisfying. Having these skills also means that patients can trust you, tell you their worries and concerns and sometimes share their most deeply held fears. It's a position of incredible trust and privilege and one that I am constantly humbled by.

I love sharing these experiences with my fellow medical students. I know we're not physically fighting in the trenches but it certainly feels like that sometimes! Being on a longer course like Medicine has allowed me to develop some firm friendships with some amazing people that are like-minded and can really relate to what it means to be a medical student: poor, neurotic, stressed, ambitious and constantly trying to hit the space between two constantly moving goal posts.

What I hate about medical school

The stress can be horrendous at times. There are times when you just feel awful. It's not a normal degree where you get 15 hours a week of lectures, 30 weeks of the year. We're talking a full-time job on the wards and study and travelling. Plus in the later years you become a member of the team and need to clerk patients, do bloods, attend MDT meetings and lots of teaching. Keeping the concentration going is tough. Add to this a consultant who just happens to feel like making you look two feet tall on the ward round, or a ward Sister with an attitude problem because you're easy prey, or getting up at the crack of dawn and travelling 20 miles to placement to be told the teaching has been cancelled and you're feeling pretty rotten.

Finally, I *hate, hate, hate, hate, hate* my student debt: just shy of £40,000. I won't write anymore because the tears that have welled up in my eyes are preventing me from seeing my computer screen...

Most valuable experience

My anaesthetics rotation at Barnsley Hospital; specifically the teaching I received from two Consultant Anaesthetists called Dr Roman and Dr Filby. Two *huge* personalities who really inspired me and taught me the fundamentals of looking after patients that are poorly.

Dr Roman would scream at me in theatre '*The Lies! The Lies! Have you heard about The Lies*?'. I had no idea what he was talking about but I soon learned 'The Lies' were (1) Morphine makes you a junky (2) Oxygen is bad for you, and (3) IV fluids cause heart failure. Dr Filby said the best thing you can give your patient is five minutes. Just five minutes everyday to assess them, their fluids, pain, chest, heart, general condition and basic vital signs. It seems so obvious but we get so caught up in managing patients that I think as medical students we forget to look after them.

Least valuable experience

I was on a surgical attachment and coming to end of a busy theatre list. The surgeon asked me to scrub in for the final case of the morning. My heart sank but I dutifully went to the sink and scrubbed up, got on my gown and returned to the operating table. The patient was present, asleep, draped and ready for surgery. The surgeon exposed the patient's penis and asked me to hold it down while he completed the operation. He took out the diathermy and in several gentle movements cut the *frenulum preputii penis* (a small band of tissue that anchors the foreskin to the penis). Operation over. '*Thank you Stephen, you can go now*'

Maybe the surgeon could see I was getting weary and wanted to involve me. On reflection I think he probably found it amusing and did it to brighten up his morning. On the other hand I suspect the scrub nurse needed a break after her four-hour marathon session at the operating table and this lesson was about teaching me the value of teamwork. I would have preferred to have just made the scrub nurse a refreshing cup of tea!

The future

In the not too distant future I will be a qualified doctor. I know that I don't want to be a surgeon and I really like the intellectual stimulation of acute medicine and delivering a baby was a real highlight of the course. Then again I loved my paediatric rotation. I like variety and so I guess GP pulls all these threads together nicely.

I never wanted to be a GP; I saw it as a soft option. However, my attachment in GP this year really inspired me and I would love to be the family doctor and build long-standing relationships with my patients. Trouble is that the NHS is changing and the role of the GP, of all doctors, is changing. I recently attended a lecture with the rest of my year group where someone from the Deanery told us that in ten years there'll be over 1,000 hospital consultants surplus to requirements but nearly 3,500 too few GP's. For someone who entered university to exercise a degree of choice, the future looks uncertain and shaped by forces beyond my control.

I want people to know that you don't have to fit into the archetypal middle-class, 17-year-old, straight A pupil to get into, and succeed in, medical school. I certainly hope you apply and if you are intelligent, committed, caring and up for the challenge then I wish you every success in the world!

Ten things I wish I had known before starting medical school

1. Facebook will become the centre of your universe. Embrace it.

2. The library is next to the union. A little more time in the library and little less time in the union and I might actually know some more medicine!

3. Turn up for placement. Funnily enough it's good for your education.

4. Don't buy all the textbooks. They go out of date and cost a fortune.

5. Enjoy medical school while you have no responsibility.

6. Say hello to at least one new person every day during Freshers' Week – everyone is just as nervous as you are.

7. Medicine attracts its fair share of bullshitters. Take it with a pinch of salt and move on.

8. The medical term for belly button is umbilicus.

9. Don't put your stethoscope round your neck until you're in the final year and even then be prepared for some abuse from the other students.

10. Learn to deal with stress: talk to friends, your family, your GP or someone who will listen. Asking for help is not a sign of weakness.

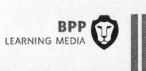

Practical Guidance Tips

Guidance

- During your first year at university buy a solid, comprehensive medical text with at least 500 pages in it. Then over the course of the first year try out shorter textbooks on specific topics to see what kind suits you. I prefer the *Rapid* series but I know others who prefer *OneStopDoc*. Try before you buy!

- Get a well-meaning relative or partner to buy you a good quality stethoscope and engrave the bell for you. This will mean that other people can't steal it from you.

- Don't buy pen torches, tourniquets and tendon hammers on day one. In fact, don't buy any of it. Get it off the medical reps.

- Do buy a good quality pair of trousers or skirt for placement and a really decent, comfortable pair of shoes.

Tips

- On their deathbed nobody looks back and says '*I wish I had been top of my year at medical school*'. Get some perspective early.

- Go on call as often as possible as a student. You learn far more in one evening than all day wandering round looking for something to do.

- Read. Read. Read. Even if its just for half an hour a day. Keeps the cogs turning and you'll be surprised how much you cover.

> 'Each year at Birmingham University, I always come to the same
> conclusion – coast as much as you can, and wing it at the end of
> the year when you have exams. Each year I am proved right.'

Name:	Neil Chanchlani
Age:	23
University:	University of Birmingham
Course:	Five-year MBChB programme
Year:	4
Extra info:	International student from Canada, intercalated in Biomedical and Healthcare Ethics (Bachelor of Arts) between my second and third year of medical school at the University of Leeds

I started medical school at aged 17. No, that does mean I was a boy genius or a modern day Doogie Howser. I came from Canada to study in the UK. In Toronto, if you were born between September and December, you got placed in the year above, whereas in Europe, you get placed in the year below.

If only that piece of information had been sent out in everybody's fresher's pack would I have avoided that question almost everyday throughout medical school.

The point is that I was very young, came from another country, and knew very little about what to expect. Some people I talked to would give me general advice such as 'medics work hard, and play harder' or some sort of cliché, but I, like you, was interested in knowing more. There wasn't a book like this available when I started medical school, but I hope mine and others' experiences can help you learn from our mistakes, and if not, at least give you a chuckle.

How it all started

I'd like to say pursuing medicine was one of those clear-cut decisions as it was for so many of my peers. Before applying for the course, many of them had logged in volunteer hours at the hospital, were interested and up-to-date with medical news, and spent their lunches in the chemistry lab doing extra work. Not me.

I was interested in science, was good at it, and that's what's probably got me to where I am today. I'm sure having a family with a medical background influenced my decision to a certain degree. Both my sisters were in medical school at the time when I was deciding, and my mom is a GP. But contrary to what others assume, I'm not sure it was a major factor.

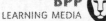

Coming from a medical background is tedious. When I was young, I used to spend hours in the car waiting for my mom while she went to deliver a baby in the hospital or be on-call. When exam season hit, my sisters were in their rooms studying for weeks on end, which was never very fun for me. Of course, any question they ever asked my mom would get met with, '*I don't know, I did it so long ago. Look it up*'; the ultimate 'advantage' of having a medical mom.

I suppose because my household was always medicine heavy, and given my aptitude for the subject, I always considered it an option. I knew it was a relatively straightforward career path that would never leave me too poor. It was nice to be seen as a contributing member of society, and although many students will pretend they don't care, it is a profession that carries status and holds a certain prestige.

Now that I've almost graduated, I often look back and wonder why I went into medicine. I think I took an easy route out. My interests at school were so much more than science; I had done English and creative writing in the hope of being a writer, and even Law and Politics in the hope of being a lawyer. The problem with those professions is that I felt (and had been warned) you had to be extremely good and skilled to get to the top. Only then would you make a lot of money and earn a decent living. That sounded tiring.

Even the most average doctor earns a decent wage and has a middle class lifestyle, why go through the trouble of being above average without any guarantee of job or lifestyle? Safe to say, I was very naive back then.

Application

I recount my application days seeming more stressful than anything else along the process. Interviews I could prepare for; look up on questions on forums, talk to others who had been through it, and at the very least, wing it on the day.

But statements, references, and forms? That is a different skill set. I didn't find it easy finding the right word to say and often felt that I was misrepresenting myself. After writing a very bland personal statement (looking back on it today still makes me cringe) and begging my biology and chemistry teachers to write me good references, I applied to Birmingham, Leicester, Nottingham, and Bristol universities.

I settled on those four universities for various reasons – academic reputation, city nightlife, size of cohort, but really it came down to where I got accepted.

I had three interviews – Bristol had rejected me as I applied for the medicine graduate entry course instead of the normal one (who wants to accept a student who can't even enter the right course code?).

To prepare, I did some mock interviews the day before with some family friends who worked in the NHS where I was brutally informed that I had no chance unless I prepared my answers better. If you think reading an article about stem cells on BBC news gives you adequate information on a 'current medical issue,' you're mistaken, just like I was.

On the day, interviewers wanted to know that I knew about training pathways, what the Royal Colleges are, awareness of ethical issues surrounding a case scenario (bombed that one in Nottingham), and that I had a natural ability to think through a situation.

It's hard remaining calm and collected in what is a nerve-wracking environment, but having sat on a medical schools admissions panel since then, it's rarely the nerves that are the deal-breaker.

The best way to assess potential candidates is to interview them, and although it is often the first time any 17-or 18-year-old has been in front of a panel, I knew that and so did they. The questions were straightforward, and it was more about getting to know that I had familiarised myself with what I was getting into rather than why I didn't get full marks on my biology exam or what the most up-to-date treatment for diabetes was.

Life as a fourth year medical student

Each year at Birmingham University, I always come to the same conclusion – coast as much as you can, and wing it at the end of the year when you have exams. Each year I am proved right.

The fourth year was spent getting to learn about specialties in greater detail; orthopaedics, cardiology, care of the elderly, etc. A great deal of time was expected to be spent in hospitals at clinics and ward rounds. A specialty block lasted five weeks, and one day consisted of medical school lectures, and one to two days consisted of hospital-based lectures. The rest was learning on the job.

Timetables are split each day so that you have an AM and PM session. We are allocated firms, which are groups of five to six people, and are expected to split ourselves up each day. Generally there are five ward rounds each week and at least five clinics going on. Students can pick and choose where they want to go, what they want to accomplish, and one person they want to go with (the best clinical partners usually get nabbed the night before via text message).

At least three to four hours of firm teaching was slotted in throughout this timetable; an hour or two with a clinical teaching fellow or registrar,

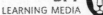

and at least an hour or two a week with a consultant. In the fourth year, the majority of our teaching was not focused on history and examination (covered in the third year), but instead on diagnosis and management.

'*What are those spots on her legs*?' and '*What surgical scar is that*?' were common spot diagnoses that we were expected to know even if we hadn't met the patient. Teachers would then spend an hour with a patient, usually with a group of five over eager medical students wanting to carry out every part of an extensive examination or asking the most inane questions irrelevant to the patient's admission, '*Is your brother a smoker too*?' It's important to be thorough, but choosing your questions and words wisely is imperative in time-restricted teaching.

All of that was in preparation for our final exams, which took place at the end of May. Nine months worth of teaching, ward rounds, book work, hospital based lectures, and medical school lectures assessed in two, three-hour multiple choice exam papers, consisting of 300 questions.

People didn't leave their house for weeks, maybe even months before those exams. You do what you need to. Some students learn better taking loads of histories and wandering the wards late night to get increased exposure, while others sit in the 24-hour library day after day memorising notes and textbooks. Both are effective, and both get you through assessments.

Social life

I didn't want to be restricted for places to go or things to do, which is why I chose to experience both Birmingham and Leeds while I'm young and can still enjoy it. Although, nowadays, my body does like to put up a fight if I go out both Friday and Saturday.

I don't think my social life suffered at all because of the course. Sure, during exam season, when you're cramming for a paper that you're due to take in two weeks, and all your friends say, '*You have loads of time...*', you do feel a bit restricted by the course load. But you can manage to go out, whether it be for drinks, a night out, a cinema trip, at least two to three times a week during the week, and both Friday and Saturday. I rarely felt the work got so overloaded that I had to stay in to catch up.

It's important to stay on top of due dates for essays or applications, but the big things to watch out for are your end of year assessments, in which case everyone in the university is in hibernation mode, and studying themselves.

Extra-curriculars are encouraged. You can often get involved as much or as little as you like, and generally, teams and societies don't meet more than once or twice a week. Almost everyone I know had joined at least one club or society, and didn't find it hard balancing work, society, and social commitments.

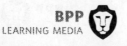

Expectations versus reality

Previously, I thought medicine was quite glamorous. My mind was moulded by television shows such as 'House' and 'Scrubs'. This led to delusions that everyone in medicine is attractive, has volatile hormones, and after all the flashy emergency surgeries, everyone heads to the bar to celebrate their successes. Ha.

As a medical student, not a great deal is required of you unless you seek it out. You can get by by slipping through the cracks, attending the bare minimum, and scraping a pass on exams. Somewhere towards the end of the programme does your status shift from medical student to trainee doctor. When that hits, you start to shape up, act more professionally, and realise the long hours, tiredness, and endless tasks will soon kick in. And there is very little you can do to prepare.

What I love about medical school

Medical school keeps me on my toes. Whether you're running a clinic, spending an hour with a patient, studying for exams, or even attending a ward round, I do often feel engaged.

You can always do something even if there's not much to do while at medical school. Because the objectives are so broad (learn everything), I never felt bored while in hospital.

Yes, your day-to-day may become routine, and you may even feel like you're constantly rote learning facts, but if I didn't enjoy doing one thing, there were always other things that I could be doing, such as working on some audit work, taking a history of a patient, or even going online and reading up on a condition.

It seems slightly disorganised, but I enjoyed being able to jump from one task to another throughout medical school; nothing required a great deal of focus. When it came to exams, you needed to know it all anyway in one sitting, so learning it that way as well seemed to work for me.

I also enjoy dealing with patients. On the ward, patients get bored and as a medical student, you have the opportunity to spend some time with them. Not necessarily to poke and prod them, but even just to have a chat with or following them up.

I learned a lot of valuable things from my patients including the different boroughs of Birmingham and what they used to be like, to the love affair one of them had with a famous footballer. Time well spent.

I found my most enjoyable moments at medical school did have to do with recovery and following a patient from beginning to end. Taking responsibility for them as a student is a daunting but rewarding role. This

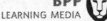

happened to me this year, and I'm bound to take even more responsibility as a final year student.

Feeling like you assisted in someone's treatment and recovery is immediately self-rewarding, and that's a guilty pleasure of the job.

What I hate about medical school

Medics (for the most part) are pretty intense. Which is probably just a nicer way to say that the large majority of them are pretty annoying as well; not as individuals, but as a group of people.

That's how a lot of people at university described medics: 'intense.' It's a unique adjective because it can refer to so many different aspects; work ethic, personality, etc. I wouldn't describe every medic I know as such, but certainly a large majority of them are.

I struggled to engage with medical students at the beginning of the course. I found them bland, obnoxious, and self-important – especially the ones who think they're god's gift to healthcare. They would say things like, '*When I'm a plastic surgeon, I'm going to work privately so I can be rich and own an Audi*'. Those are the kinds of statements where you wonder what's wrong with these people.

Of course I didn't know my entire cohort of 400, but by the end, I knew quite a few. Lots of them don't read the news, or read any books at all for that matter, and can barely hold up a conversation if the topic isn't work related. I found myself writing people off quickly.

Medical school is insular, and I felt it was important to meet and get to know as many people as possible. I have the rest of my life to hang out with medics; quite a few medics even end up marrying their colleagues! Unlike some of my classmates, I didn't negate other students' friendship because of the course they do or their background. I learnt a lot from my non-medic friends and from engaging in university societies. It would have been a mistake to let that go for the sake of chatting to someone between every lecture.

Most valuable experience

I often have teaching sessions where I come out having been ripped to shreds by the consultant for not knowing anything. '*You're in the fourth year, you need to know this...,*' often gets batted around the tiny space between me, patient, and doctor. It's moments like those that I took away from throughout my clinical years.

At first, it seems aggressive and you can get pretty worked up over how you're talked to. After a while though, you learn to take it more gracefully.

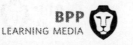

You go home and look up the disease for example, or pay close attention next time you see a patient with it. People often complain that consultants are too harsh or disinterested in medical students, but really, they do want you to learn. Sometimes, theirs or a student's attitude gets in the way of that, but I do feel that those teaching sessions were the most useful.

To be fair, I probably should've known it anyway.

Least valuable experience

I learned early that relying on medical school administration was never a good idea. I found this out when I wanted to go to the higher bodies in the medical school for straightforward requests – such as being allowed to intercalate at another university or inquire about spending my student selected component in a different specialty.

I often found them dealing with matters – whether it be telling us when our exams were, releasing grades, or even answering an email – painstakingly slowly. When met with any sort of follow up in the matter, they would raise their eyebrows, look at you confused, and your question was met with silence.

Dealing with the majority of them was tiresome, frustrating, and often inconclusive.

The future

I'd like to say that I've come out from the majority of my undergraduate medical education unscathed and ready to give up my freedom, extra-curriculars, and social life as a student to join the institution that is the NHS.

Although I do want to start earning (the debt seems endless), I am not sure I want to work as a doctor. Medicine is a great industry that lends itself to dozens of alternative careers where one need not practise.

I enjoyed medical school, the friends, and the experiences that came with it, but I more so enjoyed the academia behind it. After a couple of audit and research projects, a brief stint in a lab, and working at the *BMJ*, my current ambitions are either to enter the world of medical publishing or policymaking.

In retrospect, I probably rushed into doing medicine a bit too quickly – comforted by the fact that I'd make a decent living while working in a social, yet challenging environment. But the great thing about the course is that it gives you the expertise to do jobs where you'll require that knowledge and training but use them in a different way.

Ten things I wish I had known before starting medical school

1. Coast as much as you can. You'll get away with it, not always, but most of the time.

2. You'll probably leave studying as late as possible every year, until all you're surviving on is McDonald's and Red Bull. You'll tell yourself that you'll start earlier next year, but you won't.

3. You'll probably change specialty preferences at least once a year.

4. You will be tired. All the time. There's almost no way to combat that.

5. Always read the morning's headlines in the papers – that way you'll have something to talk to patients about.

6. Never bring a laptop to a lecture and type it up. You will forever be known as that guy.

7. If you have norovirus, you are automatically cleared for three days as sick. You can't come back into a hospital if you've had diarrhoea and vomiting for 48 hours. (Use cautiously.)

8. Your car, your music.

9. As you advance throughout medical school, the number of smokers will exponentially increase.

10. Know that at the end of the day, a job is only a job.

> 'There are plenty more careers with more money, more respect and a better lifestyle, but none quite so rewarding.'

Name:	Thomas (Tom) Kwan
Age:	22
University:	Keele University
Course:	Five-year undergraduate hybrid (PBL (problem-based learning) and lectures)
Year:	4
Extra info:	Undertook a gap year and will be taking post-fourth year intercalated MPhil in Tissue Engineering. I also got married after the second year and have never lived on campus

I'm from the group of medical students with no other medics in the family, in fact no graduates above my generation. I didn't get in first time either and subsequently know the hard times you face in deciding to place 'Medicine' on your UCAS form.

I also know how terrifying it is to pursue something you have had little contact with; and how fantastic it all seems while watching '*House*' and '*ER*'. That's the reason I chose to share my experiences, to give you just a small taste of the reality of pursuing a career in medicine.

How it all started

My journey into medicine started with something as simple as the kidneys. Studying renal anatomy in Year 9 I quickly developed a fascination with the human body, and how each individual part creates this complex 'machine'.

My interests didn't end there. The more I learnt about the normal, the more I questioned how it could go wrong. I contemplated studying the human body further with a degree in Anatomy, but I began to realise that the human body is only fascinating in the context of what it can achieve. As clichéd as it may be, I have always loved working with people, and studying the human body without the person just wouldn't fulfil my interests.

I realised that the answer lay in both the study of the healthy and diseased human body, and to work with the people in these bodies. Paramedicine was actually the first career to come to my mind, the excitement and variation appealed to me, but I began to understand that it would not give me the opportunities I was looking for. I wanted to be able to follow a patient's care from start to finish but as a paramedic I would only be involved in the presentation of the patient, and never be involved in their continuing care.

I went on to consider a career in nursing, much more hands on with patient care, but it wouldn't allow me to be in charge of that care. The opportunity to make the decisions and lead the team was what I was really looking for, and subsequently I found the answer to lie in medicine.

At the time my expectations were of a highly respected and challenging career, all about saving people's lives. I will tell you how much of that I have found to be true!

Application

My first application, at the beginning of my second year in college, went to the old universities of Edinburgh, Manchester, Nottingham and Newcastle.

I treated the application as for any job and sold myself as best I could, listing all my achievements. However after a few months I was left with four lots of 'Unsuccessful' without interview.

It took me a while to recover from the disappointment, but I became more determined and contacted the universities for feedback, resulting in my second application presenting a more mature self with further experience.

This time I applied for two newer medical schools, Keele and Hull York, and once again Manchester and Edinburgh. I was granted three interviews, the first at Keele, followed by Manchester and then Hull York. Edinburgh subsequently rejected me for a second time. The interview process is as scary as you think and I was the most petrified I have ever been.

All three followed a similar course: four interviewers opposite you firing questions one after the other: '*So why medicine and not nursing*?'; '*how do you cope with stress*?'; '*what extra-curricular activities do you do*?' etc. And they can spot a rehearsed answer instantly.

I was still recovering from the post-traumatic stress of the first two interviews when I received a letter from Keele. Only being delivered by owl could have made it more exciting. Reading just the first line ('*We would like to congratulate...*') I was soon calling everyone.

Manchester later rejected me, while the interview at Hull York was, needless to say, less stressful, and a few weeks later I received my second unconditional offer. Application to medical school is one of the most stressful things you will do, but if you are determined and can prove it, you shouldn't have a problem.

Life as a fourth year medical student

My typical day consists of time spent on the ward – anything from clerking in patients and practising examinations, to taking blood and cannulating. It's really up to us to decide what we want to learn.

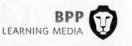

Teaching in the fourth year is diminished compared to other years. There is at least one three-hour case illustrated learning (CIL – 'advanced PBL') session a week and then two to three small seminars.

You are timetabled for two to three clinics in a week, which give the opportunity to see a large number of patients, or time in another setting such as theatre. Much of this is done in the third year, and so only makes up a small part of the fourth year. The main aim is to become comfortable with diagnosing patients and thinking up treatment plans.

Put like this the workload doesn't sound excessive but in actual fact it is by far the hardest year. Less teaching sessions makes more work at home, and to top it all off, this is the longest year of them all at 44 weeks.

Spending 9.00am till 5.00pm in the hospital is a given, but evenings and weekends are often the best times to learn. Generally a further two hours of work in the evenings and then maybe three or four over the weekend, depending on how you work, are required. And then there's the revision.

This year is the big one for us, our finals. Pretty standard for medical schools now, they are split between multiple choice questions and key feature (short answer) questions. And trust me, the multiple choice questions are harder. At this stage you are not expected to write paragraphs, simply bullet points about diagnoses and management, which is manageable if you have spent enough time on the wards.

The majority of medical schools also have a continual assessment component. Here this takes the form of case reports, which require writing a synopsis for a chosen case, and then answering questions about aspects of it such as ethics. They take a lot of time but make you consider aspects of a case normally overlooked.

Overall life as a fourth year is long and stressful, but as close to being a doctor as we have been. When you get involved in ward rounds and speaking to patients, the memories of why you started this course in the first place come flooding back, that is until the consultant asks you a question...

Social life

Never underestimate the ability of a medic to have a social life despite the massive workload.

By the fourth year, compared to other students, we are effectively graduates and, at least to me, the student union doesn't seem that appealing, but that's not to say I don't have a social life. Medicine can become claustrophobic and occasionally you just need to step back and breathe in the fresh air.

I do at least one non-medical activity every day, for example playing bass in a band, going to the gym, or just going out on the town with old high school

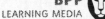

friends. Essentially medicine is a big part of my life, but not all of it. I'm a person who is doing medicine, not a medic who is trying to also be a person.

I think it's important to maintain a life outside of medicine, and to know other people who aren't medics. When you are with medics all you can do is talk medicine and you quickly forget that you know anything else. Considering I want to be in this career till I am potentially 70, I don't want to get bored of it too quickly!

Expectations versus reality

I knew medicine would be a challenge and I knew I would enjoy it, but I didn't comprehend just how much of a challenge it would be or how much I would enjoy it. I expected to be the same person but in a different stage of life, but in actual fact the demands and experiences have changed me as a person, both for the better and for the worse. Despite this, the one expectation that has not changed is this: that when I started, I would never look back, no matter how difficult it has been.

What I love about medical school

I don't often take the time to stand back and think about what I love about medical school, but I think I should more often as there is a lot I do love. My primary reason for considering this career in the first place was my fascination with the human body and my desire to learn more about it. To this end, medical school, particularly the first two years, has been truly amazing. Undertaking my first dissection of the cadavers in anatomy was one of the most truly remarkable experiences I have had and helped to further solidify my passion for this subject.

But as well as the academic side to medical school, I have found myself captivated by the more human element. I have come to love the interaction with patients and the challenges they bring. Do something right and a patient will heap praise on you, but do something wrong and they can break you down. There's a fine line to walk and it keeps you constantly reflecting on your abilities and attempting to improve yourself as much as possible and I relish this challenge.

Overall I feel I love the uniqueness of being in medical school. We are privy to some of the most personal information people will ever share and are trusted to help make their lives better. The moment for me when I knew this was a fantastic career and not your typical 9 to 5 job, was when I was stood in theatre watching the beating heart of a patient – not everyone can say they have had the opportunity to witness that.

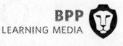

What I hate about medical school

The biggest problem any medical student will tell you is the workload. It feels as if I'm trying to complete five years of high school in one year, and then have to repeat that five times. And it just keeps on increasing. Not only do you have the work to complete from PBL, or the notes to write up from lectures, but you then also have to be consistently revising. Then there is of course clinical skills and finding willing volunteers to practise them on.

Towards the latter years you realise if you really want to get into your chosen specialty then you have to start doing some extra-curricular work, for example submitting essays for prizes, or audits and research. It never ends.

The competitive side to medicine can also seemingly amplify this workload. Not only are you trying to keep yourself afloat, but you are competing with everyone else, mostly in your own mind, for those jobs in the distant future.

One truly frustrating aspect is the medical school's ability to vastly underestimate how much pressure is on you. You will quickly get used to the comment: 'well you will have to do it when your a doctor'. That is all very well and good, except when I'm a doctor I won't also have to hold a 16-hour a week part-time job to pay the bills; when I come home at night I won't have to begin a mound of revision; I will no longer need to be part of so many committees; and the most important: I will be paid for it!

All in all I don't think there is anything I 'hate' about medical school, but there is a lot to get frustrated with.

Most valuable experience

I never thought I would say this, but my most valuable experience has been spending four weeks at a GP surgery in Year 3. As part of the third year we spent four weeks in a GP surgery to learn the workings of community based medicine. While previous placements consisted of only observing consultations, this time we were given our own rooms and our own list of patients. Of course we were not completely abandoned, and after taking an initial history and any relevant examinations, the GP came through and discussed our findings.

I was comfortable taking histories and performing examinations, but usually only after the patient had been seen and started on treatment. I was now the first person to listen to these problems and only had ten minutes to find out as much as I could.

It was a steep learning curve and as the number of waiting patients rose I learnt to hone my histories and streamline my examinations to confirm or refute my ideas. Those four weeks helped me to become much more adept at taking a concise history and performing the relevant examinations; you still won't find me becoming a GP however.

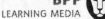

Least valuable experience

My least valuable experience came in the first year, in the form of Inter-Professional Education which sought to highlight the need of a doctor to work within a multi-disciplinary team.

Once a week students from Medicine, Nursing, Physiotherapy, Midwifery, Pharmacy and Social Work met to create a poster on a case designed to highlight our roles and how they interact. Unfortunately the process only ended up reinforcing student's stereotypes of each other. In a group of students you will always get some who do all the work and others who will let someone else do the work, and as a medical student if you try to organise the group you're just seen as arrogant by the other professions.

Perhaps it didn't achieve the desired effect as we didn't yet fully understand our own roles. In clinical years we have found ourselves naturally integrating into the multi-professional team very well, as we now have a better understanding of our roles and how the team works, by witnessing it in the real environment. There is only so much that can be achieved in classrooms when the place you will be working is on the ward.

The future

Four years ago working as a doctor seemed an age away, but now as I approach the second half of my fourth year it's very close. If anything I am more excited now than I was when I started, but it is a terrifying proposition at the same time.

There are aspects which worry me about the future, for example if I will get the job that I want, how far I will have to move for it, and what affect this will have on my plans for a future family.

Not surprisingly, considering the reasons I became interested in medicine, my current specialty of choice lies in surgery, and more specifically Plastic and Reconstructive Surgery. I do also wish to pursue academia, with a university research position, and have summarised my future like this: develop new clinical procedures in the lab; use those procedures in surgery, and finally teach them to medical students. I don't have any regrets in choosing medicine, it has provided me with the opportunities I wanted, and while it is hard, it is also extremely enjoyable.

My advice to anyone considering a career in medicine is to think long and hard. There are plenty more careers with more money, more respect and a better lifestyle, but none quite so rewarding. I hope by sharing some of my experiences I have provided you with some points that you may have never considered, and you can trust me, I'm almost a doctor.

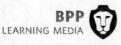

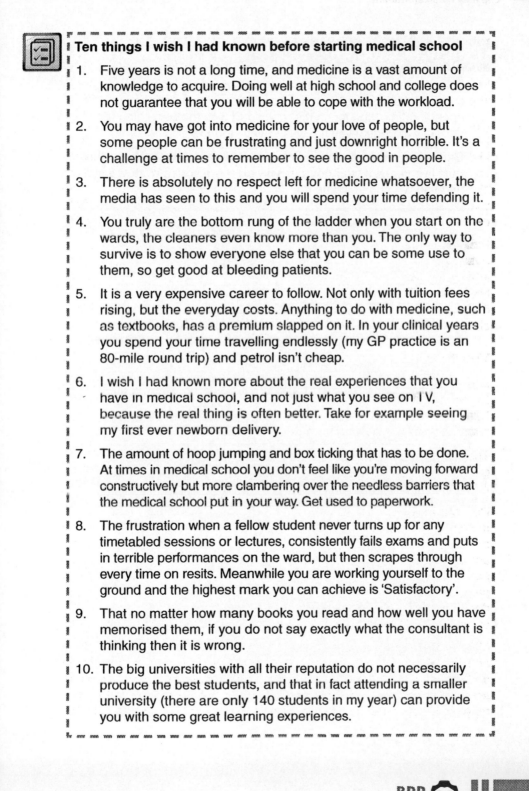

Ten things I wish I had known before starting medical school

1. Five years is not a long time, and medicine is a vast amount of knowledge to acquire. Doing well at high school and college does not guarantee that you will be able to cope with the workload.

2. You may have got into medicine for your love of people, but some people can be frustrating and just downright horrible. It's a challenge at times to remember to see the good in people.

3. There is absolutely no respect left for medicine whatsoever, the media has seen to this and you will spend your time defending it.

4. You truly are the bottom rung of the ladder when you start on the wards, the cleaners even know more than you. The only way to survive is to show everyone else that you can be some use to them, so get good at bleeding patients.

5. It is a very expensive career to follow. Not only with tuition fees rising, but the everyday costs. Anything to do with medicine, such as textbooks, has a premium slapped on it. In your clinical years you spend your time travelling endlessly (my GP practice is an 80-mile round trip) and petrol isn't cheap.

6. I wish I had known more about the real experiences that you have in medical school, and not just what you see on TV, because the real thing is often better. Take for example seeing my first ever newborn delivery.

7. The amount of hoop jumping and box ticking that has to be done. At times in medical school you don't feel like you're moving forward constructively but more clambering over the needless barriers that the medical school put in your way. Get used to paperwork.

8. The frustration when a fellow student never turns up for any timetabled sessions or lectures, consistently fails exams and puts in terrible performances on the ward, but then scrapes through every time on resits. Meanwhile you are working yourself to the ground and the highest mark you can achieve is 'Satisfactory'.

9. That no matter how many books you read and how well you have memorised them, if you do not say exactly what the consultant is thinking then it is wrong.

10. The big universities with all their reputation do not necessarily produce the best students, and that in fact attending a smaller university (there are only 140 students in my year) can provide you with some great learning experiences.

Practical Guidance Tips

- Take a year out, and not just for travelling and relaxing. Having a year out to mature, learning how to manage my money and spending time working in the real world was the best thing that I could have done, even if it was forced upon me.

- Choose a university somewhere you will be happy to live for the next five years, if your not happy living there you're work will suffer and you will soon give up.

BPP
LEARNING MEDIA

> 'Even as a medical student you feel that you are making a
> difference, even if it is just by listening to a patient.'

Name:	Kristina Lee
Age:	23
University:	University of Edinburgh
Course:	Five-year with the option to intercalate between 2nd and 3rd year
Year:	4
Extra info:	Intercalated with honours in Pharmacology

I'm Kristina currently a fourth year medic at the University of Edinburgh but in my fifth year at university as I intercalated. I am originally from Manchester where I attended a private girls' day school and I love to dance, play the violin and piano and generally have fun. I've decided to share my experiences as I love my course and I want to give you a flavour of my medical life so far and hopefully encourage others to seriously consider medicine as a career as it is exciting, fun and extremely rewarding, although definitely hard work. When I applied I didn't have much of an opportunity to speak to many medical students and so I didn't know what to expect. I therefore would've appreciated a book like this to give me a peep into the realities of being a medical student.

How it all started

I guess it sounds rather clichéd, however ever since I was young I've always wanted to be a doctor. There are no doctors in my family, so to be honest I'm not too sure where this idea came from; however I've always been fascinated by anything medically related. Sometimes I wonder whether my aspiration to be a doctor has moulded me to who I am today, for example my passion for science, desire to help people and keenness to learn, or whether it is these traits which made me want to be a doctor. Either way, I am still determined to achieve my goal and definitely feel that I made the right choice. People always ask me if the money and prestige attracted me to pursue a career in medicine and I would be lying if these factors didn't have an impact, however if these are your only motivations to do medicine, then I would quit while you can. In my opinion I can think of better ways to earn more money and gain recognition which definitely have less stress, pressure and responsibility than is required for medicine. In contrast, the job satisfaction and sense of personal achievement is definitely worth it!

Application

I applied for Medicine in my last year of school and being a 'city girl', I knew that I wanted to go to university in another city. I had a friend and a friend's brother who both went to Edinburgh and this got me thinking about Edinburgh as a potential university. However, it was only after visiting the open day, where I was not only impressed by the beautiful city but also by the course and friendly and helpful staff and students, that I knew it was where I wanted to go to. As for the other universities, I applied to Manchester as my parents wanted me to have an option to stay at home, Imperial as I felt it was the most prestigious of the London medical schools and Liverpool as it was my brother's alma mater and close to Manchester. Being totally honest, apart from these reasons, I put much less effort into picking my other choices and with hindsight I guess I didn't research them as well.

The whole application process was nerve-racking. The worst was waiting to hear from the universities, particularly as I went to a competitive school where everyone was secretly vying to get the first and most number of offers. I wasn't the first, but fortunately I had an interview and received an offer from Liverpool before Christmas, which definitely was a great relief as I knew one offer would be enough to go to medical school. After Christmas, I had interviews at Manchester and Imperial, however as I mentioned earlier, I hadn't researched these universities in any great depth so I wasn't too surprised when they both rejected me, particularly as I hadn't really prepared well for the ethical questions. Manchester's rejection was a blessing in disguise as I didn't want to stay at home, but I would be lying to say I wasn't upset. I was also gutted that I was rejected from Imperial, as they gave a great impression on their tours of the medical school at the interview and I definitely would have rather gone there than Liverpool.

My heart however was set on Edinburgh, but as they do not interview school leavers, I knew it would be a long wait until I heard anything from them. This wait was definitely the worst, especially as the rejections had knocked my confidence. However fortunately for me I am glad that it all worked out and I was offered a conditional offer which I met.

Life as a fourth year medical student

Busy! From the third year at Edinburgh the majority of teaching is clinical and based in hospitals and GP practices and in the fourth year there is a huge jump in terms of volume. The fourth year here is when you study many of the specialities such as obstetrics and gynaecology, GP, ophthalmology, dermatology, ENT, psychiatry, oncology, neurology, renal, urology, palliative care, haematology and breast. As you can tell by the long list, there is a lot to learn.

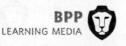

Unlike previous years, it's much harder to describe a typical day, as it very much depends on which attachment you are on, and where, as many placements are at peripheral hospitals. The year is split into three 14-week rotations, which starts with a core lecture week and finishes with exams followed by a well-deserved two week holiday. With regard to the lecture week, there is a lot to cram in, with lectures usually starting at 9.00am and, assuming the lecturers don't run over, they finish at around 4.30pm. This week, however is the most intense in terms of hours of compulsory class. For the rest of the rotation, each day depends on your attachment and varies in terms of timetabled teaching which can include ward rounds, tutorials, bedside teaching, attending clinics and theatre. It is therefore possible to have a lot of 'free' time; however in reality this time is filled up with writing case reports, reading, writing lecture notes, carrying out a research project, travelling (my GP attachment was a 50-minute drive away) and let's not forget to mention sleep, especially after a 12-hour night shift on the labour ward. The work load however is just about manageable and even though you may be in a lot of the time, medicine is very practical and you actually learn a lot from just being on the wards and from experience. Most evenings I usually spend doing extra-curricular activities, relaxing or socialising and catching up with work. It is definitely advisable to keep on top of the workload as even if you do, I still literally spend all day (from around 8.30am to around midnight) working when it comes up to exams.

Exams vary depending on each rotation but can consist of OSCEs, online MCQs (Multiple Choice Questions) and SAQs (Short Answer Questions) and a viva. Throughout the year there are also assessed case reports for your portfolio and also a research project, much like a dissertation, as well as continuous assessment of your performance while on placement. Some exams are finals and therefore are not amenable to resit exams thus requiring remedial class or resitting the year, which definitely adds to the pressure. Although stressful, I would consider the exams fair, however the lack of time to revise and the volume of information definitely makes them much harder.

Social life

The saying 'Medics work hard and play hard' is definitely true and I don't believe that medics have a less active social life because of our course, it is just important to time manage well to ensure that your work is not affected. In my first few years at university I would go out every Friday and Saturday and maybe throughout the week, however once you are in your clinical years, going out midweek isn't really feasible if you are placed in a peripheral hospital and also not wise if you have to be in the hospital the next day. This doesn't mean that we don't go out though, it just means that we make the most of our weekends and have massive end of exams parties!

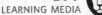

As for extra-curricular activities, medicine can be tough therefore most medics participate in some form of extra-curricular activities to have fun, relax and have a break from work. Extra-curricular activities are also crucial for demonstrating that you are an all-rounded person, much like when applying to medical school. There are plenty of opportunities to join societies, with not only the normal university clubs, but also medic specific ones which are great as everyone appreciates that Medicine is busy and therefore can have less strict commitment requirements For me, they allow me to continue my hobbies which I started before university and also to try out new things such as learning sign language. In particular, it is a great way to meet other people with similar interests outside of medicine and I have made some of my best friends from the dance society. In particular being on committees is a great opportunity to get more involved and allows you to have an input into the running of a society. This is particularly advantageous if you can ensure that the society can fit around your hectic schedule!

Expectations versus reality

To be honest I didn't know what to expect at medical school except that I knew it would be hard. I guess I was right, however, I wouldn't say it is the content that is particularly difficult (it can be sometimes), but more that the volume you need to learn is immense, which was definitely a shock. I can still remember my first day at university when we were given the list of learning objectives which was the same length as all the syllabuses for my A level courses combined and thought this was certainly manageable, until I realised that these were only for the first semester! Before starting university I always thought that getting into medical school would be the greatest obstacle to becoming a doctor, however now I'm not so sure. Getting into medical school is clearly a crucial step to becoming a doctor, however once you're in it is definitely tough and just as competitive, if not more. Even though I knew that fellow medics would be clever, it is definitely true when people say medics are the crème de la crème. You may have been the smartest in your year at school, but at medical school it is a completely different league and it can often be a shock when you realise this is no longer the case, which can sometimes be difficult to adjust to.

What I love about medical school

Genuinely, I love almost everything about medical school and there definitely isn't enough space here to discuss it all. Not only is the content of the course extremely interesting but also the variety it brings. Even though our timetables are very busy I enjoy that we don't sit in lectures all day and we have the opportunity to meet new people and work as part of a team in the hospital. I find the science of medicine extremely

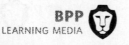

interesting and in particularly I love the mental stimulation of working out diagnoses and management plans (albeit less tricky than in *'House'*). The opportunity to carry out practical clinical skills and procedures are fun and satisfying, however most of all I enjoy interacting and communicating with other people. As a medical student, we are very fortunate to be able to talk to patients, who often confide a lot of personal information to you. You often learn a lot from patients and even as a medical student you feel that you are making a difference, even if it is just by listening to a patient.

During my time at medical school, I've also made a lot of wonderful friends – people who have the same interests and aspirations as me and have the same passion for helping others. There is definitely a sense of community and camaraderie between medics and everybody understands what you are going through and can offer an enormous amount of support at times when you need it. My experience so far at Edinburgh has been amazing – it's a brilliant course with great friends set in a beautiful city with a lot of history and things to do. What more could I ask for? (ok, so there are maybe a few things– see the next section).

What I hate about medical school

Without a doubt medical school is hard and can be extremely stressful, especially leading up to exams. The sheer volume of work and limited time adds pressure to an already demanding course. For example a 14-week rotation may sound like a long time, however if you imagine that within this time you have to learn three systems such as dermatology, ENT and ophthalmology, which are by no means small; carry out a three-week GP attachment with a case report to write and consultations videos to make and also conduct and write up a research project, you can see that 14 weeks is definitely not long enough. However, if that isn't tight already, there is also no study leave before exams with teaching finishing on the Friday and exams starting on Monday. Now if I told you that this rotation is considered the 'easiest' of the three in the fourth year at Edinburgh, I hope you get an idea what I mean by the sheer volume of work.

The competitiveness of medics is another thing that can be annoying, although to be honest I am also guilty of this myself. If you thought getting into medical school is competitive, once in it only gets worse. The competition is not a bad thing, no one (or very few people) are there to 'back stab you', instead everybody is trying to boost their CVs, which adds to the pressure of doing well while also carrying out extra-curricular activities and additional research just to keep on par.

However even though we can have long draining days, short holidays which don't really give you much time to recoup or earn any money and have less time to go home and visit our families, I guess this is a reality of medicine as a career. On many occasions I have wondered why I chose to put myself through this and why I didn't pick something less stressful, however overcoming these moments has made me stronger and more determined to become a doctor.

Most valuable experience

I guess for me intercalating was one of my most valuable experiences. Not only did I learn about a subject in depth and make new friends, but I also developed a lot of skills including critical appraisal, presenting and statistics, which are all applicable to medicine. Intercalating also helped me learn a lot about myself during this year. In particular I realised that I had definitely made the right choice with choosing medicine as my career path and intercalating also opened my eyes to research, which before I definitely thought was boring and geeky! Intercalating also made me appreciate the close relationship between medics and I feel very privileged to be part of such a close-knit community.

Least valuable experience

I don't think I can pinpoint anything that I would consider my least valuable experience. Everything I have done during my time at medical school I feel I have learnt something and no matter how small I would still consider it important.

The future

My ultimate goal is still to become a doctor and even though I'm in my fourth year, I still feel I have a long way to go. Since starting my clinical years I have only properly started to appreciate the vast number of specialties on offer and I guess for the first time I am not too sure what I want to do. I am however keen to do surgery, but I also want to have good work-life balance, especially as I do one day want to settle down and have a family. Therefore at the moment ENT seems very attractive not only because of the mixture of the medical and surgical conditions, the variety of operations from simple to radical surgeries but also as there is a large proportion of out-patient practice. I am glad however that I do not have to decide just right now. In ten years' time, I hope to be on track to becoming a consultant, which in these days is getting more competitive. Maybe I'll be a registrar, doing an MD or PhD or working abroad for a year, who knows, but I hope I will still be pursuing my dream. I definitely have no regrets and I feel medicine for me was the right choice. My advice would be to do something that you enjoy, therefore even if it is difficult along the way, it will be worth it for the sense of satisfaction and achievement.

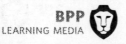

Ten things I wish I had known before starting medical school

1. Enjoy your time with your family and friends at home, as there is definitely less time at medical school.

2. You will no longer be a straight A student, getting a B is already considered very good!

3. Brush up on computer skills. Most non-practical exams are done on the computer, so it's good to make sure you are competent at typing.

4. You can have a life outside of medicine – work is not everything. Remember to have fun.

5. Make the most of your holidays, particularly to save money as in the later years as it gets very expensive.

6. You will be fine without a TV.

7. After starting medical school, you realise that you know so little.

8. You will be bombarded with questions from your non-medic friends and family asking you to diagnose them.

9. You will suffer from medical student syndrome (have a look on Wikipedia).

10. It is ok to moan about your course and feel sorry for yourself around exam time. Medicine is hard so try to ignore the comments when people say, 'Well, you chose to do medicine!'

Practical Guidance Tips

- Go to the university open days and speak to the teaching staff and medical students. Don't be shy to ask them questions as they can give you the best insight to what their university is like and format of their course and I guess for those applying they can give you a lot of information regarding their application procedure.

- Don't rush into buying textbooks. Try to suss out which ones you like – go to the library, borrow from your friends or ask older years. It will save you a lot of money.

'It's an absolute privilege to meet and spend time with patients day-in day-out.'

Name: Ross Kenny
Age: 23
University: University of Nottingham
Course: Five-year BMedSci BMBS
Year: 4
Extra info: Keen scuba diver hoping to one day use medicine to work and dive around the world

I am currently in the fourth year of a five-year undergraduate medical degree having arrived here following grammar school and a quite wonderful gap year. Unlike many of my peers, I don't come from a medical background – neither of my parents are doctors, nor do any of my friend's parents have any claim on the world of healthcare. So pursuing a career in medicine was for all intents and purposes, a gamble. For all I knew (*and perhaps hoped*), it was '*Scrubs*', '*ER*' and '*House*' all rolled into one.

I want to share my experiences of medical school thus far, as I remember just how foreign it all seems when sitting on the other side of the application process. Therefore, without further ado, here is my insight into Nottingham Medical School and my life as a medical student.

How it all started

I first thought of becoming a doctor during a careers meeting at school. I wasn't very good at art or languages; my strength lay in the sciences and so inevitably the first course shoved under my nose was 'Medicine'. However, after looking at the requirements, the countless A*'s required and various other hoops to be jumped through – I'm ashamed to say, I thought I'd look elsewhere!

I first applied to study Law. To this day I don't know why, and I quickly came to the conclusion that I would make a terrible lawyer. I studied Maths, Biology and Chemistry at A level and secretly enjoyed them. So I embarked upon a gap year to decide what to do with my life. After encouragement from my parents and former school teachers, I decided that maybe six months of 'jumping through hoops' for a career spanning 40 years wasn't a bad trade off. I gained as much work experience as I could shake a stick at, took the UKCAT and rolled the UCAS dice.

A lot of people worry about coming up with a clever response as to why they want to study medicine. To me it was obvious. You want to study medicine because you want to become a doctor – it's a means to an end.

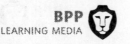

The real question is why do you want to become a doctor? When I was 18, I remember my over-riding desire was to do something that *never* got dull or boring. From an outsider's perspective, that certainly seemed to be the case with medicine. Not only is every specialty constantly evolving and improving but the problems within them evolve too. There will always be a conundrum; a problem that cannot be solved. That is why medicine stood out above all else. Oh, and the prospect of delaying any more career decisions for another seven years didn't seem like the end of the world either!

Application

I decided to apply to Birmingham, Nottingham, Newcastle and Southampton. I didn't fancy doing a PBL course, and London looked too expensive to me, so I opted for good universities, in good cities, that I felt I had a chance of getting into. My first choice was Nottingham, but this was mostly due to the university and not necessarily the course. The campus at Nottingham in my opinion is second to none and I really enjoyed the open day. Being from Birmingham as well, I knew it wasn't too far from my local washing machine and bank manager (mum and dad respectively).

I remember at the time feeling a curious mix of nerves and cautious optimism. I knew I had the grades and a good UKCAT score but was unsure if I had enough work experience. I had left school by this point and wasn't keen on the idea of a second gap year. My first response was a rejection from Southampton. I remember well the sinking feeling when I opened the webpage and saw '*unsuccessful*', but a few days later I received letters from the other three universities inviting me to come for interview. I felt incredibly excited; it was all becoming a reality. My first interview was at Birmingham. A quick tour around the school before experiencing an awkward hour in a waiting room nervously smiling at other candidates, wishing them luck… but not too much! I was interviewed by a psychiatrist, a member of the faculty and a medical student. They asked me lots of questions about career pathways; what happened after medical school, F1/F2 etc. They were friendly, asked politely about my work experience, what I had learnt, and why I wanted to come to Birmingham. A nice start.

Next up was Newcastle. I visited a friend and stayed the night before, and consequently went out to watch the football and experience what Newcastle had to offer. The interview however was not so enjoyable. The interviewers were nice enough; I was more the product of my own downfall. When asked if I was interested in research, I replied positively. When they asked why, I was not so quick to respond. In truth, I didn't really know what medical research entailed; I just thought it sounded good. It didn't.

After missing my train for the interview at Nottingham, I felt that it wasn't going to be my day. Fortunately, the ticket collector for the next train failed to notice my incorrect ticket (result!) and I made it to the interview in the nick of time. Another token tour around the school and before I knew it I was sat in front of a doctor and a head teacher from a local school. They asked me what I thought made a good doctor (empathy!) and if I thought I had the appropriate qualities. They asked me what my friends would say about me as a person; so after suppressing all the insults and rude remarks I'm sure they would say, I told them that I'd be recommended as honest and hard-working. Finally they asked me all about my gap year and travel plans; in truth it was a really nice chat.

I was accepted into Birmingham soon after my interview. I remember feeling overjoyed, ecstatic that all the hard-work had paid off – I was going to med school! In the New Year I found out that I had been accepted to Nottingham and so accepted the place without hesitation, despite not having heard from Newcastle... probably just saving another rejection letter!

Life as a fourth year medical student

I don't know if a 'typical' day exists as a clinical-phase medical student, as it varies so much depending on which placement you're on. Normally you're expected to be in for at least 9.00am and the days are roughly split into morning and afternoon sessions, finishing any time between 4.00pm and 6.00pm. Sometimes you have on-call shifts through the night (and loads of fun!) or on weekends (not so much fun!) You get a good mixture of clinics, theatre sessions, ward-based work and structured teaching, often in groups of five to ten.

On average, I would say you're in the hospital for 25–30 hours per week, with a few sessions designated for 'private study.' The rest of the time is your own, but in truth a fair amount of this is taken up by background reading, especially close to exams! Exams are usually in January and June, but in the fourth year they are in November and May and final fifth year exams are taken in February. There are coursework elements to most modules, consisting of an essay or case-based discussion however the vast majority of your assessments take place in online-exam format at the end of a given module.

The workload is definitely manageable although it may not seem like it during exams. Medical students can appear encumbered with work, but the truth is there's just a lot to learn. Medicine is a fact-based discipline and while there are concepts to understand and methodologies to learn, the key to success in exams is being able to take on board a large volume of information.

Social life

Nottingham University has an excellent social set-up and without this I don't know if undergoing the rigours of medical school would be possible. In the first and second year, which are mostly lecture based, you can happily go out two or three nights per week to a host of different bars and clubs, finances providing. In clinical phase, it's not acceptable to be around patients while hung-over, and you wouldn't want to be stuck in a hot theatre room the morning after a big night out. It's all about time management and not letting work get on top of you – you learn quickly to make the most of your evenings and weekends!

The social scene isn't all about going out either. There are more clubs and societies to be involved in than there are hours in the day. There are a wide range of sports clubs, new theatre, musical productions and lots of charity work to get stuck into, making the whole university experience one to cherish.

Expectations versus reality

I can honestly say that I had no idea what to expect from medical school prior to university. It was obvious that there would be a lot of work but I expected to have my head buried in textbooks and spend all of my time in the library. In reality, the course at Nottingham has kept inline with technology and provides lots of useful resources on-line. Lectures and articles are uploaded daily, which allow you to work from home in comfort.

What I love about medical school

There are many great things about being at medical school, but if I had to choose the aspect I love most of all, I would have to say that it's the people you meet that make it so special. First and foremost; your colleagues. I'll admit that I was nervous about what other students would be like – we'd all fought so hard to get there and competitive people aren't always easy to get along with. However, four years down the line I can safely say that the medical students I've come across may well be driven and competitive but are also honest, friendly and tend to have a great sense of humour. It's not all about work – it's about enjoying the overall experience and getting through the hard times together. This camaraderie is highlighted brilliantly with hundreds of medical students each year becoming involved in the production of the medic's musical, not to mention the numerous sports teams and societies that meet throughout the year.

Doctors tend to love to teach and so they're a great resource to learn from. They are intelligent and on the whole have good people skills hence the opportunity to shadow them throughout the clinical years is really beneficial. This is true for other healthcare professionals too, such as nurses and midwives, who are often very keen to help medical students learn.

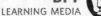

Finally and most importantly, it's an absolute privilege to meet and spend time with patients day-in day-out. As medical students, we examine patients, take up their free time gathering histories, practise taking blood and putting in cannulas, and perform other uncomfortable or intimate procedures on them. Yet throughout all of this, patients do not complain; they're so accommodating in aiding our learning and really want to help us as much as we want to help them. Each individual patient has their own story to tell and tells it in their own special way; it's this uniqueness to each patient that makes medicine so engaging and worthwhile.

What I hate about medical school

Hate is a strong word, but there are definitely aspects of medical school that could be improved. For example, sometimes placements can seem like an exercise in gathering signatures to say that you've attended this clinic or that theatre and thus you can't actually appreciate what's going on. Not earning any money can also be quite difficult to manage. The loans enter and leave your account like passing ships in the night and at times it can be a real struggle. You have to get yourself to different hospitals in quite a large catchment area; at Nottingham we can be placed in Lincoln, Derby or Mansfield, all at a considerable travel cost. Another aspect of that is the fact that bursaries and other financial aid is mostly means-tested against your parental income, which isn't a fair reflection of the financial support you receive. The silver lining to this grey cloud is that the NHS covers your tuition fees in your final year!

Another hard truth that really can't be avoided is working to a different schedule to your non-medic friends. While your friends are celebrating graduation, you will be revising hard for your exams. If you asked most medical students if it was worth it, I'm sure they'd agree that it's a fair trade.

Most valuable experience

My most valuable experience was delivering a child at the beginning of the fourth year. It is well documented that childbirth is truly unbelievable but being hands-on in the delivery room was a breath-taking event. It was around 2.00am during the middle of a night shift in Mansfield. A woman progressing well through labour with her fourth child was happy for me to assist the experienced midwife. The midwife appreciated my enthusiasm and attempts to calm the mother. Before long, both parties agreed to let me take charge... under the watchful eye of the midwife of course! It was incredible; as though three years of hard work and countless exams all paid off in one moment. The delivery was uncomplicated and everything went well. The next day I visited the mother with her new born and chatted for almost an hour about the whole event. Just to be a part of something so major and to feel like I

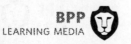

was partly responsible for the successful outcome put everything into perspective. It reaffirmed to me that there's nothing else I'd rather do.

Least valuable experience

In all honesty, I found lectures – the medium through which most content is delivered in the first two years, filled with 320 other people – more distracting than beneficial. There are some brilliant lecturers and some really interesting topics but often it's hard to focus! In the clinical phase it's completely different; the emphasis is on individual learning or small group tutorials which cover the vast majority of the content, making it easier to recall when revising. It must also be said that the medical school tries many approaches to learning in lots of different ways: seminars, practical sessions, cadaver dissection and ward based teaching to name but a few.

The future

I'm excited to progress through my medical career, with becoming a junior doctor only a matter of months away. I've always been optimistic about life as a doctor and four years down the line this hasn't changed. My understanding of the complex world of the NHS and career pathways has improved somewhat but I'm still unsure as to where I'll end up. I'm happy with that.

There are pros and cons to any career; for instance I love the flexibility and potential to retrain in different specialties. I hate the fact that I'll have to work on Christmas Day some years. It's true that it is hard work and long hours but so is anything worth doing and why should medicine be any different? I still firmly believe that it is a brilliant profession that I am proud to be training to be a part of one day.

It is definitely true that you can be influenced by the people you meet and this has happened to me to a certain extent. I have worked closely with a consultant anaesthetist who gave me a real insight into anaesthetics that I very much enjoyed. I've also assisted surgeons in theatre and would love to pursue a career in a surgical specialty. Hopefully in ten years' time I'll be on a training programme in a specialty I love, working hard towards becoming a consultant. Finally, I would love to practise medicine around the world as each healthcare system has something new and interesting to offer. All things considered, I know that I made the right decision and am excited for my future.

To all those thinking of applying, I wish you the very best of luck in your application and future career.

Ten things I wish I had known before starting medical school

1. NHS employees including medical students get 20% off at Nandos and Subway. Carry your ID badge always.

2. Don't buy textbooks; borrow them from the library for free.

3. Don't be afraid to say 'I don't understand'.

4. You will never find a pair of scrub shoes for theatre that fit you. Get used to it.

5. You don't need to buy every piece of kit offered to you in the first month of medical school. Relax, you can always borrow one.

6. Think about getting a piece of work published or presented before your final year.

7. Try to do an audit at some point during the course – ask a consultant and they'll usually have an idea.

8. Doctors no longer wear white coats so nip that dream in the bud.

9. Offer midwives cups of tea… without them having to ask.

10. Just because you have a MacBook doesn't entitle you to bring it everywhere.

Practical Guidance Tips

- Try to stay calm in the interview and don't pretend to know something you know nothing about, just because it sounds good. Honesty is the best policy!

- Don't worry too much about the work-life balance at medical school; you will find your happy medium and what works best for you!

Chapter 5

The final year: A dose of reality from five medical students

Zuliana K Banda

Thomas Wood

Ban Sharif

Douglas H Blackwood

Sheetal Patel

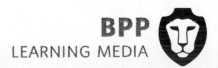

BPP
LEARNING MEDIA

The final year: A dose of reality from five medical students

'What doesn't kill you only makes you stronger'.

Name:	Zuliana K Banda
Age:	31
University:	Newcastle University
Course:	Five-year MBBS
Year:	Final
Extra info:	Mature student with previous BA (Hons) degree in Social Policy and Politics

My journey into medicine began three years after I graduated in Social Policy and Politics from the Royal Holloway University of London (RHUL). Today, aged 31, I am in my last fight to gaining the title 'doctor with a big D'. This however, is my second attempt, thanks to a disastrous MOSLER (Multi-station Objective Structured Clinical Examination Record) exam for which I will spare the intricate details. In short, while my peers celebrated their entry into 'real' medicine in the summer of 2011, I on the other hand, spent it wishing that karma would someday soon enough catch up with the fiend (examiner) who caused my demise. After going through a conveyor belt of emotions, from anger, guilt and pain to just feeling numb, I finally came to accept that sometimes the unexpected happens and life moves on. I have had to pick myself up (including my pride), dust myself off and keep on stepping! And so here I am, sharing some of my experiences. Perhaps my story will inspire someone to 'keep on stepping' even in times of adversity.

How it all started

My story is rather simple and lacks the glamour and embellishment of stories commonly shared by medics about what led them into medicine.

Following numerous stints in unfulfilling, mind numbingly boring and worst of all poorly paid – in short, unrewarding jobs – I found myself yearning for a career that was interesting, fulfilling, challenging and importantly, *well paid*. Being a graduate as it turned out was not all that it was cracked up to be! After months of 'soul searching' and 'career researching', I seemed to have discovered my calling to medicine and my life started to move in the right direction. I felt an inexplicable sense of peace.

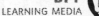

As if to check my own resilience for a future career in medicine, I got a weekend job (in addition to my normal 9 to 5) as a nursing auxiliary at a private nursing home. This experience truly and profoundly encouraged my personal growth and facilitated an informed insight. Compassion, empathy, enthusiasm, tolerance and stamina are all so needed in the caring profession. I enjoyed interacting with the residents and assisting with daily activities. Occasionally, I would be frustrated by my lack of medical knowledge, especially when I had to care for people with chronic illness. However, what I didn't know then only fuelled my desire to attain a comprehensive understanding of the scientific basis of disease and illness. I became more determined to become a doctor someday.

In September 2005 I enrolled on a ten month 'Access to Medicine' course at the College of West Anglia, King's Lynn. This intensive course brought me up to scratch with the basic sciences, as my A levels and degree were non-science based. I met people from varied backgrounds, but we all had one goal in common: *to get into medical school and eventually become doctors!* This experience was an eye-opener into life as a medic. It is then I understood that I was entering into a highly competitive and pressured field, with an interesting mix of characters, ranging from annoying, inconsiderate, egotistical, to the more likeable, friendly, reserved, compassionate personalities, and sometimes a confusing mixture of everything!

Application

In 2005, I applied for Medicine to Newcastle University, St George's University of London, the University of Aberdeen and the University of East Anglia (UEA). I did not have a 'plan B', it was now or never.

I picked Newcastle after being persuaded, by an acquaintance studying there, that I had a good chance of getting in. As fate would have it, following a very brief interview, Newcastle was the only medical school to offer me a place on the condition that I passed the Access course with distinctions. As you can imagine I was ecstatic when I did! So the moral of the story is never give up!

I applied for the fourth-year graduate course at St George's, mainly because I wanted to stay in London. However, to secure an interview I was required to sit the GAMSAT exam in the first week of January 2006. In hindsight, this was an unrealistic target, considering I had only been on the Access course for three months. But as the saying goes, 'where there is a will there is a way'! Undeterred, I sat the GAMSAT realistic in my expectations, that the pigs had more chance of flying and doing somersaults in the air than I had of seeing the interview rooms of St George's. And so, armed with a pen and pencil, an eraser and a calculator

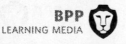

and a rosary firmly around my neck, I proceeded to the exam hall. With my head held high I sat at my designated desk and spent the next five hours in total academic oblivion, and before I could say 'medicine' the exam was over. Slightly shaken but certainly not stirred, I walked out of the exam hall just as I had walked in, without too much expectation!

Aberdeen rejected my application without interview. By this point I was too happy with my offer from Newcastle to even care! UEA rejected me after interview. Having grilled me for over 35 minutes on why I wanted to study medicine and other things which I cannot remember for the life of me, they decided I was not their cup of tea and needless to say, the feeling was mutual.

In the end, the gain outweighed the pain (of writing personal statements, dreadfully waiting for acceptance and exam results). Alas! My dream was *not* deferred and my life had just begun!

Life as a final year medical student

Final year this time around is less daunting as I know what to expect. I have completed three-week attachments in Paediatrics, Psychiatry, Primary Care (GP), Obstetrics and Gynaecology and Preparation for Practice (P4P). I have less than 16 weeks in Medicine and Surgery before exams.

My typical day starts at 6.45am and ends at 5.00pm. I literally fight with my alarm pressing the 'snooze' button at least five times before I actually get out of bed! By 9.00am I am either in an outpatient clinic or on a ward trying to get competencies such as catheterisation and cannulation signed off. On average I attend three seminars / lectures per week. These are usually interactive and involve group presentations / discussions of various clinical cases and sometimes clinical skill practise. Having a car has helped immensely as sometimes I start my day at one hospital (35 miles away) and end it at another (four miles away).

Surgical days start earlier at 8.00am. Opportunities sometimes arise to scrub up in theatre and if you are really lucky you even get to hold a limb or an instrument (note the sarcasm). Most times one ends up assuming the medical student position in the 'loser' spot somewhere in the far distance away from the operating table, avoiding questions at *all times* as this often ends up in humiliation.

The work load can be overwhelming. However, it *is* manageable providing you 'work smart' and don't get caught up in the small detail. I spend roughly two to three hours per day studying either at home or in the library and longer at the weekends.

Clinical assessments carried out at the end of each rotation normally by a consultant follow the same format as the final year MOSLER exams.

They last approximately 25 minutes and include observed history taking and examination of a relevant system, plus a ten-minute grilling on the management of the patient. On the whole, these assessments are a useful tool for measuring progress, however, because they are quite subjective they can be misleading. Professionalism is also assessed at the end of each rotation and basically involves a simple tick box of whether or not you have attended and have been a 'good boy or girl' (ie not killed a patient or strategically run over an annoying colleague in the car park!).

Social life

My social life in Newcastle is almost non-existent! There just never seems to be enough time; with pending deadlines for assignments, job application forms and study time, the list goes on! I will try my best to make up for lost time after finals! In all honesty, having gone through the whole 'drink-party-club' sequence (with a T-shirt to show for it) during my first degree, I do prefer a quiet night in than to go out on the '*toon*'. Occasionally, I do enjoy a nice meal or coffee with friends and in recent years have attempted a few nights out clubbing, which have invariably ended up with me playing baby-sitter to one or two intoxicated friends. Not that I am complaining! I also attend a local gym regularly, and find that keeping fit helps lift my mood, re-focus my mind and keeps me energised.

Another reason for my lack of action on Newcastle's social scene is that most of my friends live down south, so I only ever get to let my hair down in the true sense when I go to London to visit family and friends, mostly during term breaks.

Expectations versus reality

I have acquired knowledge and developed a wide range of skills far beyond my expectations over the last five years. I laugh when I think back to some of my memorable experiences in earlier years. For example, failing to put a blood pressure cuff correctly on a patient during an OSCE (Multi-station Objective Structured Clinic Examination) in the first year and feeling, and no doubt, looking completely stupid! I have also matured during this process, learning about how I react to and cope with stress, recognising my strengths and weaknesses, to discovering my love for surgery.

Like in all walks of life, it would be naïve to assume that prejudice does not exist in medicine. People either choose to ignore it or accept it. In the past I have found myself trying to rationalise my experiences. For example being blatantly ignored during teaching sessions as if I were not present (despite almost literally popping my eyeballs out of my head just to get some much needed eye contact from the tutor), I sometimes wondered if they (including some students) literally could not see me or if they *chose* not to see me?

What I love about medical school

I love that medical school affords me the unique opportunity and privilege to connect with people in ways that I otherwise wouldn't. Witnessing some life changing moments can be a humbling experience that helps puts life into perspective. For example, being present when a patient is told they have cancer, you can't help but share the patient's grief or when a woman delivers a baby, you celebrate in her joy. I am always reminded about my past experience in the nursing home, how empathy and compassion are important qualities to have as a doctor.

I love that once in a while you come across a rare species of special and amazing doctor, who inspire you to be the best you can be! For me it was my elective supervisor Dr Soka Nyirenda (AKA the deity of medicine!), a consultant physician at the University Teaching Hospital in Lusaka, Zambia. I was in awe of his depth and breadth of knowledge, his effortless ability to break down the most complicated concepts to basics, his unique, witty, probing style and importantly his compassion towards people. Nyirenda undeniably made teaching appealing and learning interesting. I learned not to be content with simply knowing 'how' but to strive to understand 'why'. Ward rounds were always entertaining, as everyone from students to registrars anticipated being 'wired' (asked questions). Nyirenda would often mock saying '*doctors with a small D... I can see you are all getting cyanosed especially as the questions get hotter towards the end of the line!*'

I enjoy being in the theatre environment, scrubing up, standing next to the surgeon and feeling a sense of belonging, wishing secretly that time would fast forward so that I can be the one doing the cutting and suturing!

Finally, I appreciate the fact there is always someone else willing to give the most stupid answer or ask the most stupid question that everyone else secretly wants to ask but usually don't just to avoid looking like complete fools!

What I hate about medical school

One of the most annoying things about medical school is not medical school itself. Rather it is the self-appointed people who love the sound of their own voice and spend a lot of time arguing endlessly over trivial details (wasting everyone else's time) during seminars / tutorials. To make matters worse they are worryingly delusional about the supremacy of their contributions to any discussion! They also tend to be the chronic over users of the word 'surely'. Yes… 'surely' what they have to say has got to be far more important than anyone else in the entire universe!

Like most students, I hate the stress and pressure of deadlines (ie foundation job application, assignments).

Filling out those countless feedback forms after each teaching session can be a bit tedious. By the end of the day, one just ends up writing single words... 'good', 'ok' or 'borderline'!

Most valuable experience

My elective in Zambia, apart from being the only time I will ever get to doss *legitimately*, was a great learning experience. Impressed by the sheer enthusiasm, passion and commitment of doctors to teaching combined with seeing patients' in dire poverty with real healthcare needs, I knew I had to return and contribute positively in the near future.

During the third year, I was given the opportunity to be a co-author on a paper about anticoagulants which was later published in a peer reviewed journal. This was my first experience writing a scientific paper. It was quite challenging in that I had to read and appraise many research articles and prioritise my time between work and university. By the end of the project I had gained invaluable knowledge not only on the topic itself but also in the publication process. For example, the paper was initially rejected and then accepted and then we had to rebut the reviewer comments / suggestions. This amazing experience opened doors to more writing opportunities with two additional publications on thrombectomy devices and peripheral vascular disease.

Least valuable experience

One of my least valuable experiences was my third year paediatric rotation under a particular consultant who spent half of his time telling us about the importance of basic principles, so much so, that he forgot to tell us what those basic principles actually were! Needless to say, by the end of the four-week rotation after learning absolutely nothing, except that 'basic principles are important', I was glad when the rotation ended! I remained to remember that basic principles are indeed important, whatever they are!

The future

'What doesn't kill you only makes you stronger.' This has become my reality. Having to re-do finals has been emotionally and psychologically challenging to say the least! Over the past few months I have come to realise that I am stronger than I thought I was. My hopes for the future are to become a doctor (with a big D!). I do not have another option. I firmly believe at this moment as I am writing that I will make it. I look forward to working and earning a wage and importantly to being happy, whatever the circumstance!

From this experience I have learnt that life is *not* a bed of roses, rather thorns and bees are always lurking in the midst... one just has to be prepared for the sting! Success is learning to cope with the unexpected then stepping forward and taking charge with the goal still firmly in sight!

Ten things I wish I had known before starting medical school

1. It is called the 'growth hormone' *not* the 'growing hormone'!

2. Medical school is full of blaggers and they all come in different shapes and sizes and inevitably you will become one too.

3. It is not always what it is cracked up to be.

4. Sometimes silence speaks volumes.

5. The nurses really do run the hospital, be nice or they will eat you alive!

6. Don't be surprised when people say hello to you one day and completely blank you the next. You cease to exist when their posse are around... accept and move on.

7. Psychiatrists really are mad... but interesting!

8. You will be humiliated not once, not twice... this is just part of the process.

9. You will meet amazing people, embrace them when you do! They will make all the difference to your experience.

10. Don't be afraid to stand up for yourself, you don't suddenly cease to have feelings and rights when you become a medical student even if your seniors think so.

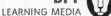

Practical Guidance Tips

- Make sure you have a strong support network of family and friends. Medical school can be tough. You really have to be mentally prepared and develop a thick layer of skin pretty quickly.

- Don't get caught up in believing your own hype. Stick to the 'basic principles' of humility, empathy and patience and you will be just fine.

- Know your anatomy! This will help you immensely!

'The standard answer to the interview question 'why do you want to be a doctor?' is 'because I want to help people'. They're lying. Deep down they want to be heroes.'

Name: Thomas Wood
Age: 27
University: Oxford University
Course: Four-year Oxford Graduate Entry Medicine
Year: Final
Extra info: In my spare time I run, coach rowing and run a circuit training class for clinical medical students. I also watch a variety of American medical dramas, which is basically like free revision

I am a graduate medic doing the four-year 'fast-track' course at Oxford. I graduated from Cambridge with a degree in Natural Sciences (Biochemistry) in 2007 and went straight into my medical degree.

How it all started

I first thought about medicine towards the second year of my degree. I pretty much had a fourth year Masters in Biochemistry already arranged, with a view to a PhD and heading into academia. While I did enjoy the subject, it suddenly struck me as a largely futile career in the grand scheme of things. Some people do research for the pure love of knowledge, but a typical biochemistry career path looks like this:

1. Spend three years in a PhD trying to get bacteria to express a protein.

2. Spend x number of years crystallising your protein as a post-doc.

3. Spend five years as a lecturer characterising your protein's structure with various imaging techniques in order to determine just what it does and how.

4. Spend 20 years as a professor teaching bored / boring students about your protein.

5. Look back on your life and realise that nobody cares about you. Or your protein.

Now, I won't pretend that medicine is particularly glamorous. The first 15 years involve a lot of jumping through hoops and then, once you convince someone to let you be a consultant, you drown in paperwork and admin. However, it struck me as the perfect way to apply the basic physiology

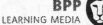

and biochemistry that I found very interesting to the real world. I haven't ever regretted the switch. The standard answer to the interview question '*Why do you want to be a doctor?*' is '*because I want to help people*'. They're lying. Deep down they want to be heroes. Yes, sometimes you work 100-hour weeks (don't tell the EU), but nobody signs up to be a doctor and expects to work 9 to 5 their whole lives. You also do a lot of boring dogsbody work, as you would in any job when you're bottom of the food chain. However, there's nothing quite like the feeling of doing chest compressions in a pool of blood or (for the less adrenaline-driven) having a patient send you a thank you card for a job well done. It's totally worth it.

Application

When I applied to graduate entry courses I had two main criteria:

1.   Not in London
2.   No expensive / lengthy entrance exams

I was in the middle of my final year and I didn't have time to study for a GAMSAT or equivalent. I also hadn't seen the allure of London yet, and didn't think I could afford the capital living costs for four years. This left me with Oxford, Cambridge, Liverpool and Birmingham. Applying as a 'graduate', I was slightly more used to the application process, so it wasn't as nerve-wracking as I remember from my first UCAS days. Despite having straight first-class marks at Cambridge, I was rejected without an interview. This had been my 'safe' choice, which they probably figured out. I also missed my interviews to Birmingham and Liverpool because I had already had an offer from Oxford by then and knew that was where I wanted to go.

The Oxford interviews were held over two days. You now get assigned a college, but back then you picked two and got interviews at both. My main college was Pembroke, where I got one 'science' interview based on stuff I knew from my degree and work I'd done in labs over the summer. There were also questions about the changing face of the NHS careers, so anyone interviewing must always be informed on the current state of medicine. The important thing is to have an opinion and always appear engaged. I also had an interview based on ethics and why I wanted to do medicine. Please don't say '*to help people*'. Have an interesting story about yourself and be honest. I've done a lot of mock interviewing for future applicants, and my main advice is to have a smile on your face and be enthusiastic. It really is that simple. You have to remember that these people have to teach you for four to six years, and if you have a nice 20-minute chat in your interview then they know you'll be a good student.

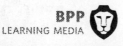

Life as a final year medical student

As a grad medic at Oxford, you spend the first year doing pre-clinical medicine. In the second year you join up with the normal fourth years but have extra lectures and exams to catch up. After that, you're all together for the fifth and sixth years. The way Oxford runs its final year is fantastic (not that I'm biased at all)... The only drawback is that your 'holiday' between the fifth and sixth year is a long weekend.

The final year started with six weeks in general medicine, which I really enjoyed. However, it's essential that you become part of the team. Most consultants expect you to disappear to the library, but you should know what patients you have on the ward and what the plan is. I would usually spend three to four hours on the ward in the morning with the team. The students split the patients and presented them on the consultant ward round, so I went in a little early on those days to swot up on mine. This is also a great time to learn some acute medical skills when your team is on take. You'll get to see the strokes and pneumonias that will be your bread and butter once you're pounding the wards as a house officer.

Surgery doesn't really do it for me, so my six weeks in breast / endocrine and colorectal were more relaxed. At this point I took more time off during the day to relax and do a little work. It's good to find yourself a registrar or consultant who likes to teach and spend a day or two in clinic and theatre with them. My main advice is to turn up and wave at the patients in the surgical admissions lounge in the morning. It varies greatly, but most old-school consultants won't let you near the patient if you haven't met them before.

I then had three weeks' holiday before 12 weeks of 'specialties' and DGH (District General Hospital) before Christmas. If you get a holiday in the six-month run-up to finals, make use of it. You'll need it before the real work kicks in. Those last three months are all about balancing time in the hospital with time to do book work. I spent maybe two hours a day in the hospital to practise examining patients and seeing some interesting conditions. I won't pretend that I was in the library the rest of the time. I planned to put in a hard two months before exams and wasn't too worried about work – I just kept it ticking over.

The best thing about Oxford is the teaching in the final year. There are almost daily teaching sessions that use cases to work through the whole syllabus. These are repeated three or four times, so you can just drop in when you have a free hour. There are also sessions using 'Harvey' – a programmable manikin where you go over most of the basic life support, ECG and cardiovascular examination skills you'll need. This is topped off with an intensive two-week lecture course right before finals that covers all the basics and goes over a number of past papers. Finals happen in early February. I'll let you know how they go...

Social life

The most important thing you can do to keep sane during a long intensive course such as Medicine is to have hobbies. In my first two years there was a reasonable amount of free time because we were expected to study the basics of medicine on our own. This meant that I had time to row for around 20 hours a week and see my friends. In the first year I didn't do much work at all because all the basic physiology and biochemistry had been covered in my first degree. Those people who had done Psychology or Chemistry had to spend a little more time in the library! In essence, you can do pretty much anything you like outside of medicine; you just need to find time to do it. Get up early to do sport or work and then give yourself time off in the afternoons. Being a part of a society or group can be really good for your CV. My job interviews focused quite heavily on teaching, and while I had spent time teaching younger medical students, I largely talked about my experiences coaching rowing, which was really relevant.

Expectations versus reality

I had no specific expectations when I started my training, and I think it's best to go into it open-minded. Lots of people who do the full six years get a bit bored of the basic sciences, but keep your eye on the prize. Our patient contact started almost immediately, which made the hours of book work constantly worth it, because you wanted to be informed enough to understand what you were seeing in the clinical setting. However, you need to remember that you are essentially a useless parasite. Don't turn up expecting people to teach you at the drop of a hat. They have a stressful job to do and you are not a priority. Conversely, if you turn up early and are polite to staff and as helpful as you can be, people will always make time for you.

What I love about medical school

Being a medical student is a brilliant carte blanche to experience pretty much anything you want. I don't think I used it quite enough, but you can turn up anywhere at any time, explain who you are and almost always get a good reception. Senior doctors love having students who are keen and well informed. If you're keen, you can see some really cool stuff in clinic, assist on big cases in theatre and help with trauma / crash calls in resus. Everyone's experience of medical school is completely different, and this is largely to do with being in the right place at the right time. You'll never be able to guess when the good stuff will happen, but being around when things go south means that you have great stories to share with your peers. Then you can make them jealous because you were the one that got to put a central line in.

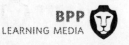

What I hate about medical school

This is probably the section where people will complain about the hard work and long hours. Boo hoo. If this worries you, close the book and apply for Media Studies. As a doctor (even more than as a medical student), you will work long hours for no recognition until you specialise. Embrace it. The long hours in the library or on the delivery ward waiting for somebody to give birth so you can get your log book signed are all good experience for the real world.

What I hate about medical school are medical students. Not all medical students, obviously, but there are a reasonably large group of them that will make your life a chore. Medicine attracts a certain type of personality that is desperate to be loved and craves attention. They will steal all the jobs on ward rounds and hoard books and notes. They will answer first in lectures and will always have self-important opinion about everything. These are not the people who come top of the year. They just annoy everybody else and burn future bridges as they strive to become 'the best'. I did very well in both my degrees, but it wasn't for a lack of helping others or sharing the workload. Remember that almost all of your peers will be perfectly good doctors and if you work together, getting out of med school alive will be much easier. I was more than happy to share my notes with my friends, and then when I got down to the wire and hadn't covered a topic for an exam, the favour was always returned. If you want to build your CV or learn / see something specific, there are continuous opportunities that don't require you to work at the expense of your fellow students. Medicine is a team game, and if you play it as such, it's so much more fun!

Most valuable experience

About a month into medical school, we were on a ward in Milton Keynes. A consultant surgeon crammed ten of us around a patient and kindly (but firmly) told one of us to examine the abdomen. We'd barely read it in a book, let alone knew what to do in real life, but he looked at me and up I stepped. I haven't sweated that much in my entire life. I did most of it wrong, but that's not the point. This situation will happen every day during clinical school, so the sooner you just have a go, the easier it gets. The feedback you get from examining patients with seniors is some of the best teaching you'll get.

Least valuable experience

Being attached to urology in my first clinical year. Arriving on the ward, there was an extensive programme of clinics, theatre lists and teaching handed to us. Hardly any of it happened. Consultants had no time to talk to us, and we were generally very unwelcome. I'm still not sure why this was the case, but it happens. It's important to persevere and

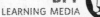

make sure you get the teaching you need, but if that doesn't happen, don't punish yourself. I watched a lot of daytime TV that month.

The future

One frustrating thing about medical school is that I still don't know what I want to do with my life. I've never regretted changing careers, but I couldn't even tell you if I want to be a surgeon or a medic. Many people know what they want to be the minute they step through the door and can't wait to specialise, and that's great. The thing I am wary of is the long and competitive training pathway into most hospital specialities, and this is something everyone should take into consideration. The starting pay for doctors isn't bad, but it doesn't go up very quickly until you're a consultant. Unless you want to be a GP, you have to accept that you'll work most of the hours in the day until you're in your forties. At this point I have no qualms about that, but you never know how your situation will change in terms of job prospects, partners and family life. I fully intend to become a consultant within the decade, with an MD or PhD along the way, but in terms of what area of medicine, who knows!

Ten things I wish I had known before starting medical school

1. Boys – shave your face and iron your shirt. This may sound obvious, but not everyone does it. Patients will respect a well-presented doctor, and some consultants have been known to send home students who don't look professional!

2. Share notes and find a work buddy or buddies. People you can bounce ideas off, sound like an idiot around when you get stuff wrong and practice examinations on. As I said above, whatever you can do to reduce your personal workload and that of your friends will pay dividends when it comes to the big exams.

3. Remember that you can revise anywhere. You'll learn more doing practice questions with a mate in the gym, or discussing topics over dinner with friends, than you will by bashing your head against books in the library for hours on end.

4. You're an adult. If you get to a point where a four-hour clinic is dragging and you can't stay awake, politely excuse yourself. If you're not learning anything valuable, your time is better spent elsewhere.

5. Don't take it all too seriously or expect certain things from certain people or certain rotations. Sometimes it's best to just go with the flow – remember that this is all experience for a 40-year career.

6. Make yourself useful as early as possible. If you turn up on the wards with no skills, you're basically just getting in the way. Practice putting in cannulas and taking bloods in the skills lab before you start clinical rotations. The best thing to do is borrow some kit and have a go on your friends. Just don't tell anyone I told you that. This way you can take the load off the house officers, giving them more time to teach you.

7. Enjoy your time off. Be lazy once in a while. Many people worry that they could always be doing more and learning more, but that will never stop. Being relaxed and well rested when things get stressful will reduce the amount of time you spend silently weeping.

8. Don't expect everyone to teach you. Some doctors are rude or stressed or both.

9. Don't take it personally. It's easy to get jaded when you constantly come up against people who aren't helpful. If you feel you're not getting anywhere in a certain rotation, tell the medical school. This is also a good time to secretly take a few days off and not worry about it!

10. Be nice to nurses. This is a lesson you can't learn early enough, and will be valuable your entire career. Nurses are lovely on the whole and will make your life so much easier if you are polite and helpful. They know a lot more than you do, I promise. As a student, always ask the nurse in charge before seeing a patient of theirs. Look down on them at your peril.

Practical Guidance Tips

- In summary – be polite, useful and don't take it too seriously. Medical school is really good fun.

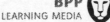

'You're responsible for your own success.'

Name: Ban Sharif
Age: 24
University: St George's, University of London
Course: Five-year MBBS programme
Year: Final
Extra info: Intercalated BSc from Imperial College London

I am the middle child in a family of five; my older brother did not want to do medicine so I thought I'd give it a go! I went to medical school straight from high school. Medical school didn't just teach me medicine, but also how to live independently and has made me the person I am today. I have decided to share my personal experiences in this book because there really isn't enough out there about what it is like in medical school. There is plenty on how to get into medical school but nothing to tell you what you're really in for. Of course each person will have their own experience and there's nothing to say you will have the same experiences but you may relate to what I have to say and consider things you hadn't thought of.

How it all started

I can remember back to when I was five years old living in London, walking with my father to a small newsagent five minutes away from our flat. We passed some parked cars and my father paused and stood by one (a Mercedes) and said that if I got into medical school; he would buy one for me. Of course medical school was the last thing on my mind – what use was a car to me? I would much rather he bought me chocolate. As you can tell, medicine has always been a big feature in my family, my parents are doctors; and coming from an Arab background as far as careers went I had a lot of choice. It was either medicine or engineering! In all seriousness though, while my parents inspired my decision I was not pressured into it. As time went on I realised I had an aptitude for science, more so than maths and humanities based subjects in school. That together with the fact that a career in medicine is respected well paid, and 'international' and secure helped me make a decision. I still find it difficult to explain why I chose to study medicine. I don't have an amazing, inspiring answer: I didn't know what else to do. A lot of other medical students and doctors I have asked surprisingly say the same thing. I toyed with the idea of studying dentistry instead but last minute decided to stick to medicine.

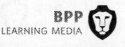

Application

I had to leave London when I was 14 because my father got a new job. I was not happy. So when it came to applying for Medicine, I was determined to go to a medical school in London. I applied in September 2004 to four different medical schools in London: Imperial College London, University College London (UCL), King's College London (KCL) and St George's, University of London (SGUL). I had to take the BMAT to fulfil the entry requirements for UCL. I was invited for interview at UCL and SGUL. I got straight rejections from Imperial and KCL. I had my interview at UCL first and I was so happy to have finally heard something from a university. By this point, all my friends who had applied to other degrees had a few offers already and all I had got was a postcard / letter confirming my application had been received. So, I certainly felt anxious and stressed. Looking back, I was not prepared for this interview. I remember being ill at the time too. The interview itself was awful. I was asked vague questions and was challenged on a few things I had written in my personal statement. As I came out and talked to other candidates, it became clear that the interviewers had already made up their mind about some candidates and this was reflected in their questions. One potential medical student said he had only been asked 'why medicine?' and that was it. I received my rejection in the post promptly after that fateful day! My interview at SGUL took place a few days later. After having practice being interviewed at UCL, I was a lot better prepared for SGUL. I felt at ease instantly and I thought the questions were fairer. I received my offer the following evening. I was really happy when I logged onto UCAS Track and saw I got an offer. While I was disappointed with my three rejections it didn't matter that I only had one offer because at the end of the day, I only needed one offer to have the opportunity to study medicine. In terms of the application process as whole, I would not say it was a fair process. A level students applying to medicine are of a high standard, some even higher. They can all potentially fulfil the entry requirements and then some. I can understand that it is difficult to differentiate students from each other but BMAT; UKCAT etc are not necessarily the best way to do that. Also what people managed to do in their gap year / travels because they had the opportunity to do so does not mean that they will make better doctors than those who didn't.

Life as a final year medical student

The final year at SGUL according to the now 'old curriculum' was divided into six rotations: assistant house officer (AHO) in Medicine, AHO in Surgery, general practice (GP), Emergency Medicine with Anaesthetics, Public health with interprofessional practice (IPP) and finally elective. According to the old curriculum, written finals were sat at the end of the fourth year. By the final year structured regular teaching did not take place. There weren't any lectures taking place for the whole year simultaneously as in previous years.

The year started for everyone in the same way. We all had to undertake a two week 'course' called 'advanced clinical practice 'or 'ACP'. This was made up of talks in the morning aimed at preparing us all for life on the wards as junior doctors. There were various workshops in the afternoon centred on the same thing. The most useful thing I took away from these two weeks were talks and workshops aimed at preparing us for the annual UKFPO (United Kingdom Foundation Programme Office) application and its white space questions.

After ACP, I went to a district general hospital for five weeks for my AHO Medicine rotation. AHO meant shadowing the house officer (ie Foundation Year 1 doctor) and doing tasks and jobs that a house officer would be expected to do. It was also a time to hone existing communication, examination and practical skills learnt over the previous five years. My day typically started at 9.00 am with a ward round and the rest of the day was spent doing jobs. I usually finished around 5.00-6.00pm. There was regular teaching a few times a week by junior doctors which was useful. I occasionally did on calls / nights with an FY1 doctor. In terms of assessment for this rotation, I had to present a case to my consultant and discuss management. At the end I had to get an attachment certificate signed and graded by my consultant and FY1.

My next rotation was AHO Surgery (Urology) at a busy teaching hospital. I usually had to be there before 8.00am and my day would typically last until 6.00pm. Again, the day started with a ward round and the rest of the day doing jobs with the option of going to theatre to watch / assist in some operations. There was some ward teaching by doctors. With this rotation, I got to supervise more junior medical students. Again, the assessment and sign-off for AHO Surgery was the same as for Medicine.

My next rotation was general practice. I spent five weeks at a practice in Croydon. I started at 8.30am and finished for lunch around 1.00pm. Then I usually had a three to four hour lunch break interspersed with accompanying the GP on home visits. Clinic would start again at 4.00pm and go on until 7.00pm. I then did anesthetics and emergency medicine. At the end of this attachment, there were two exams. Following this, I did a five week public health and IPP (see least valuable experience) attachment. Public health consisted of two weeks' of lectures / videos and workshops. The assessment consisted of a *'Dragons' Den'* style presentation selling a particular public health intervention in the country where your elective will take place. Exams took place early June and consisted of three OSCE days. In the two weeks prior to exams, we had

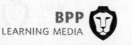

revision lectures scheduled, which were useful but by that stage you should already know it all!

Social life

As a final year student I had a more active social life than in previous years. With written finals out the way, I did not feel the need to study every night like I had done in the past. I was going out a few times a week. It was not always like this, in the third and fourth year, my attachments were a lot busier and I would limit social activities to once a week – including extra-curricular activities eg society meetings / events. It is possible to have an active social life as a medical student regardless of the year you are in. You just have to work out early on where your priorities lie eg if you're ok with just passing then you can afford to go out a lot more – you also need to be organised and clever about how you manage your time. Extra-curricular activities can also take up time. I was involved with Amnesty International Society at SGUL, it was a great way to meet new people and also organise events centred on things I was passionate about. I even got to go to a U2 concert – for free, courtesy of Bono. It is important to be a part of at least one society, even if just for a short while because of the people you meet and also to feel that you have been a part of something successful. Not to mention that it looks good on your CV and possibly in foundation applications in the future.

Expectations versus reality

I always knew medical school was going to be tough and challenging but I never imagined what it would involve. All I had to go on was a few days' work experience and a few weeks volunteering at a hospital. Making that leap from complete novice to doctor was a difficult one. I was not prepared for the endless lectures, clinical skills sessions, anatomy teaching in the dissecting room, heavy emphasis on communication skills, endless attachments, my unhealthy attachment to the Oxford Handbook of Clinical Medicine and the not-so-wonderful OSCEs!

What I love about medical school

- Elective: it may be a long wait but to be able to go to another country for a period of time to experience medicine is a wonderful opportunity. It may change your life.

- Friendships: when you're in a place for so long with the same people, you start and cultivate friendships which can act as a second family. There can be a real camaraderie between medical students, even those from different years.

- No essays! This is probably heavily dependent on the medical school you go to but unlike other degrees, there is a distinct lack of essay writing and assignments involved. It really is just learning and memorising a large volume of information.

- Clinical years: finally you get to learn the useful stuff! You finally get to witness what medicine is really all about on the wards, you get to see real patients, take blood, and you get to learn about all these diseases you have only heard snippets about.

- Ample opportunities: to do research, to win a prize, to have a publication or two, become president of a society or the medical school itself.

What I hate about medical school

- Length: I disliked the duration, made even longer with an intercalated BSc. Yes, it does pass by quickly but it can also drag. It's no fun saying you're still a student well into your twenties when your non-medic peers have been working for a good few years.

- Competition: this is fierce and will take place from the first year. You will compete daily amongst your friends on how many lectures you've been through, how much work you've done, grades, prizes, on ward rounds / ward work. Medicine is incredibly dog-eat-dog and sadly everyone is in it for themselves. On the flip side, competition drives you to work harder (just keep it healthy!).

- Arrogance: arrogance may exist from day one for some people – it's just in their nature, however medical school is a breeding ground for arrogance and even the humblest soul may succumb to it.

- Pre-clinical years: I did not enjoy these. They consisted largely of daily, relentless lectures which centred on medicine on a very molecular level. Yes, it is useful but you do not really get to experience medicine and learn about the endless clinical conditions until third year.

- Dissecting room: this was not for me. I could never get my head around dissecting a dead body. I had no problem in theatre but I could not bear the dissecting room. It smells awful (you will end up smelling of formaldehyde all day), it is unpleasant and I think there are other ways of learning anatomy if you're not that way inclined (eg anatomy books!).

Most valuable experience

My most valuable experience was my elective. I finally got the chance to experience medicine in another country and focus in depth on what

I may want to do in the future. I have always considered moving to America because my family live there and it is a great place to be a doctor. It was also my first time flying alone and living in another country by myself. I went to Los Angeles. It was great seeing the contrasts between the NHS in the UK and private healthcare in the states. The sunshine did not hurt either! This experience has made me consider sitting USMLE exams and potentially pursuing a career in America.

Least valuable experience

IPP: a three week attachment in final year where I had to talk to other healthcare professionals about the multidisciplinary team and the interactions between each member. Three weeks was far too long for this and it was a completely unnecessary exercise because you get to learn about the multidisciplinary team while on the wards between eg physiotherapists, occupational therapists etc.

The future

After being a super keen medical student who practically lived on the wards, I decided that ward based medicine / surgery was not for me. While I enjoy it, I think there are too many uncertainties in medicine; it certainly is not like it is in the books – which at times I find a little frustrating. I think the hours and degree of stress in a medic or surgeon are great and at times the correlation between hours and pay do not match up fairly. I have decided that radiology is for me, I enjoy it immensely, the lifestyle is great and it is an ever expanding field (and yes, I do like the idea of sitting in the dark all day, staring at a computer screen). Jokes aside, another question I get asked from people when I tell them I want to be a radiologist is: 'won't you miss the patient contact?' Funnily enough, no, I don't think I will. And that's ok because there are lots of specialities within medicine which do not involve patient contact. I would also like to work in America at some point – either temporarily or indefinitely. In ten years' time I see myself being a radiologist – where? I'll leave that to fate.

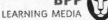

Ten things I wish I had known before starting medical school

1. Five or six years is a long time. After being in education for so long, you are let out into the real world as a very young 23/24-year-old! You feel a few years behind your non-medic peers and you can't help but wonder where all the time went.

2. Doing an intercalated BSc is a total waste of time. A lot of people sit on the fence about this and say it may help you when it comes to specialty applications. Ok well, I'll tell it to you straight. Do not do it! (Unless you have to as part of your degree).

3. It does not prepare you for being a doctor – until you have full responsibility for a patient and are held accountable, you just don't know what it is like.

4. Don't make enemies / fall out with anyone. Five or six years is a long time to be avoiding people, facing hostility and holding grudges. Plus, the medical world is small – you may end up working in the same hospital some day!

5. I did not realise before I started medical school the amount of public speaking and communication involved. If I had known the sheer number of presentations, role playing and general 'talking' involved, I would have thought twice! Fortunately though, being forced to do those things from the first year made me more at ease at public speaking and it became very easy as the years went by.

6. Work hard from day one. It will pay off. Make yourself stand out academically – it is the only thing that consistently matters. Get some distinctions under your belt.

7. It does not matter what medical school you went to, you're responsible for your own success.

8. It will push you to work way beyond any limit you thought you had. The competition between your peers alone will drive you to study all day (and all night).

9. You may often find yourself wondering if you're good enough / up to it / capable on a regular basis, especially when there are so many other high achievers.

10. I should have done Dentistry!

Practical Guidance Tips

- It is normal to feel like you want to quit several times throughout medical school. People often do. Don't be hasty. Find someone to confide in, dust yourself off and start again.

- (Unofficial) entry requirements for medical school: thick skin, self-confidence and determination.

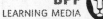

'University is simply the best experience that anybody can have and I do truly feel sorry for those people who miss out.'

Name:	Douglas H Blackwood
Age:	25
University:	University of Glasgow
Course:	Five-year MBChB (PBL – problem-based learning)
Year:	Final
Extra info:	Intercalated BSc (Hons) in Philosophy, Medicine and Society from University College London

Despite having now adopted the embittered air of the perennially delayed Londoner I was actually born and brought up 500 miles to the north in a 'new town' on the outskirts of Glasgow called East Kilbride. Finding it very hard to appropriately describe the place where I have spent the majority of my life I turned, as in all such times of ignorance, to that bastion of knowledge, 'Google', in order to find some words of wisdom from a more poetic mind than mine. Perhaps George Orwell, who spent time there while recovering from TB, had mentioned it in his memoirs or maybe Lorraine Kelly, who is also from East Kilbride, had described it during an interview.

However, type '*famous quotes East Kilbride*' into the search bar and what you find is a list of quotes for taxis, removal vans, coach hire, clutch replacement and many more. And it is perhaps this, rather than simple prose that best sums up my home town; it is, in essence, a practical as opposed to a romantic place. There may not be any particular reason for anybody to journey there, but at the same time, and as Google's extensive list of available services proves, there really isn't any need to leave it either.

And so it was here that I spent the best part of my formative years as a fairly happy and contented child. I attended my local primary school, moved on to what Alastair Campbell would describe as a 'bog-standard comprehensive' and then drudged through the various exams and application forms that took me towards university. Of course along the way there were the standard trials and tribulations of being a teenager. Everyone goes through an awkward phase at some point and I was certainly no different. I look back at photos with bleached blond hair and Harry Potter style glasses that are quite frankly cringeworthy. But on the whole I am very grateful that the largest problem I had was when bouncers stopped accepting a 'European Driving License' as valid ID.

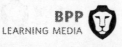

How it all started

Good question.

Thinking back, I really don't know how or when I decided that I wanted to be a doctor. From an early age it was what I was planning to do although the reason escapes me. My mother was hospitalised with an auto-immune illness for a short period when I was very young so perhaps it was this that convinced me to 'help the sick'. On the other hand my father was made redundant when the steel-works were closed down in the early 90s, so perhaps it was the more selfish promise of a steady job and solid career that persuaded me. Perhaps it was neither. And since I don't plan on spending a few hundred pounds discussing it with a psychologist we will probably never know.

What I do know is that when you get an idea into your head it takes a lot more effort to challenge it than to accept it. And in truth that is why I continued on this path. On occasion I considered whether medicine was the correct career for me but never with enough conviction to change my mind. After all what would I do instead? At that point in my life I really could only think of law or medicine as possible future careers.

Looking back I think this was partly due to poor career guidance at school but I too must take responsibility for lazily falling back on my assumption that I would study medicine. In retrospect I at least wish I had been aware that there were other choices open to me and that I didn't have to pigeon-hole myself into a life-long career at 16 years old; that I could have studied a non-practical course such as history or politics at a top university and that there would have been jobs and opportunities at the end of it. To anybody who is in a similar position I would simply mention that if you are smart and hard-working then you will be successful in whatever field or job you choose.

Application

It has been a long time now since I filled out my own UCAS forms. And it seems that over the last decade things have become a lot harder, with ever-increasing competition for a limited number of places and additional hurdles such as the UKCAT for people to jump over. I certainly don't envy the applicants of today and if I'm honest I think I would struggle to be accepted if I was applying in 2012.

In Scotland the exam structure means that we sit our main exams a year early and therefore you have already met the exam requirements before applying. As such it is purely your personal statement and interview that determine if you are accepted.

I was fortunate in having a teacher whose daughter had recently applied to medical school and who took me under her wing when writing my personal statement. The help of somebody who had an understanding of the process was invaluable and I doubt I would have been successful without her.

When applying I chose the four Scottish medical schools; Glasgow, Edinburgh, Aberdeen and Dundee. There was no anti-English sentiment I must point out but purely a practical consideration given that English universities had recently started charging tuition fees.

Out of these, Edinburgh rejected me straight away. Aberdeen offered me an interview but a Travelodge fire-alarm and evacuation at 3.00am somewhat dented my performance and I was promptly rejected. The Dundee interview was very pleasant and seemed like more of a chat than a formal process while Glasgow was a more traditional and nerve-racking experience of sitting in a dark room with two senior doctors and a tape recorder. Looking back I am unsure exactly how I managed to win a place at Glasgow as I was woefully unprepared. The only questions I can remember were ones that I blatantly did not know the answer to; firstly on the cause of Down's syndrome and secondly on why I felt the PBL course would suit my learning style (at this point I'm pretty sure I didn't know what PBL stood for let alone meant). It seems having all the answers isn't an absolute necessity but I still suggest that you read up on the type of course the university has and on any recent medical stories in the news.

Life as a final year medical student

After six years of medical school, six years of lectures and labs, six years of wards and hospitals, in the end it all boils down to just a couple of days. Two three-hour written papers on a single day and 50 five-minute OSCE (practical) stations spread over four days. The thought and the fear of this is what dominates every day of your life for the months leading up to it.

The day starts with a flitting visit to the hospital where I am supposedly completing a placement followed by a dash to the library for hour after hour of studying. It is of course important to show your face at your hospital and you can certainly pick up bits and pieces that will help you but in truth it's the time with the books that will get you that pass. After a few hours going over notes it is generally time to scour the SL (this stands for study landscape and is Glasgow Medical School pretension for library) in search of people with whom to head to Byers Road and grab something to eat. A pizza from 'Little Italy' or a pasta from 'Papperinos' provides some energy but also a much needed break from the monotony. After that brief moment of respite it's a chance to hit one of the many past papers that get passed around between students (these are invaluable) and find out if any of that knowledge is sticking around for long enough to make it

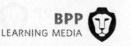
BPP
LEARNING MEDIA

worthwhile. At the back of 11.00pm I pack up my bits and pieces and head towards the subway ready to do it all again tomorrow. As I walk through Ashton lane it seems a tad more raucous than normal. That's right, it's Friday night. Well, at least I don't have to go to the hospital in the morning.

Social life

This is the reason to go to university. University is simply the best experience that anybody can have and I do truly feel sorry for those people who miss out. It may be a cliché but it really is a time when you get to try new things, meet new people and have experiences you wouldn't previously have considered.

In particular the first few weeks after you start is the best time to meet new people. I think everybody is a little scared when they start university, especially if you don't really know anybody. But you soon find that everyone else is in the same position and your 'no-friends' predicament forces you to go out of your way to chat to people.

Of course exams and study weigh heavily on your mind but the truth is that even if you are studying medicine, which takes up a significantly greater amount of your time than other degrees, you still have a gargantuan amount of free time when compared to when you start working.

And if you go to Glasgow you are in a great place to enjoy it. The university is in the heart of the West End with a plethora of facilities literally on your doorstep. Walk down to Byers Road between lectures and grab a coffee at 'Tinderbox', an independent chain which produces arguably the nicest coffee you will find. When you're finished for the day you can head to Ashton Lane, a small street packed with bars that is only a stone's throw from the medical school. And for those nights when a couple of pints isn't quite enough you have the choice of two separate unions, 'classy' establishments in the West End like 'Viper', or you can jump on the underground and head into the city centre for dozens of different clubs.

The other thing to mention is that it's definitely a good idea to get involved in as many different clubs and activities that you can from the outset. Whether its rock climbing or politics you will find other people doing things that either you already love or just want to try for the first time. When I was at Glasgow I didn't fully get involved with things from an early stage and it is definitely one of my biggest regrets. Fortunately when I moved down to London to do my intercalated degree I learned from this mistake and got much more involved.

Expectations versus reality

I have no doubt that medical school was very different from what I expected, although I couldn't for the life of me tell you what it was I did expect. I think that the whole experience of university from the sheer volume of things that you learn to the experiences that you have mean that you change dramatically during this time. This is particularly true for Medicine simply because the course lasts so long. The person that you are, or who you think you will be, when you are 17 or 18 is a million miles from the person that you emerge as at 23 or 24.

What I love about medical school

Overall medical school is a wonderful experience.

First, from a purely practical point of view, when you successfully finish your degree you walk into a relatively well-paid job as a matter of course, and there are few other degrees that you could say that about in the current economic climate.

Second, you are at university for either five or six years and this does allow you to enjoy the full university experience for at least two or three years longer than others. I can't even imagine finishing university after only three years. I really only felt that I was starting to get to grips with the whole experience by the third year and that the final three were where I really got to enjoy it.

It is also the point where you will be most free and have the greatest amount of control over your life until you retire. When you are at school there are scheduled classes and teachers chasing you up for missing them. When you are at work you are being paid to show up and people are relying on you so you have to be there. But at university, while of course it is important to attend your classes (and I am not advocating not doing so), the truth is that you are effectively responsible for your own learning. If you choose to skip a particular lecture then the only person that will suffer is you and this gives you a great deal of flexibility. If you want to sleep until 11.00am and then study until midnight then that is your call. If you are having a particularly stressful day and want to chill out for a couple of hours and get a coffee then that is your decision. Being a student gives you a large amount of responsibility over yourself and your own life but it gives you a freedom that you lose when you start working and have a responsibility for other people.

What I hate about medical school

Medical school is not like a normal degree. At the end of the day there is simply no way of getting around this fact. In regards of workload, free time and exam stress it is on a completely different level to 'normal' degrees.

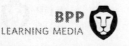

During medical school I was fortunate to have been able to complete an intercalated degree at UCL in Philosophy, Medicine and Society. During this we were parachuted into second and third year classes of a separate degree and worked with students who were studying towards a BSc. Each week I generally had around six to eight hours of classes with the rest of the time free for reading, writing essays or more accurately having fun. In medicine it is likely that you will work six to eight hours a day and you will do your own additional studying outside of this. This is not including the fact that your terms will generally start earlier and finish later. You can certainly try to pack in as much as you can (and you should) but in the end you will not be able to enjoy the social side of university quite as much as people doing other degrees. Unfortunately I have all too many memories of walking past the Queen Margaret Union and through the bars of Ashton Lane seeing my fellow students drinking and laughing while I made my way to the library prior to exams.

Another, more philosophical point, is that unlike other degrees there is no pursuit of knowledge for knowledge's own sake in medicine. When I was at UCL I had a professor who told me that studying didn't always mean slaving over a book in the library but that going for a walk or a coffee and using that time to think was equally as important. This sort of attitude does not fly in medicine. Studying is working in the truest sense of the word.

Most valuable experience

It is July 2005 and I am sitting in Palma airport with a group of my friends. We have just had a 'lad's' holiday in Magaluf and it is now time to go home. Now the end of a holiday is invariably a bad time for anybody but in this instance it is made significantly worse by the fact that I am the only person going home. Everyone else is going to be enjoying the sun, sea and the other, less wholesome, activities of Majorca for another week. This early flight home has been brought about by the fact that two months earlier I managed to fail my first year exams. Now, as can be seen by the fact that I booked a holiday at the same time as the resits, this came as somewhat of a shock to me. I don't think that prior to this I had failed an exam since Biff, Chip and Kipper were looking for the magic key. All other exams from Standard Grades (GCSE) to Highers had been pretty straightforward. A couple of weeks of studying prior to the exam and then a nice comfortable A or at worst a B if it was a bit tricky. But here I am, sitting on a budget airline home beside a particularly large chap and a baby in order to resit an exam that if I fail will mean my expulsion from medical school. These experiences are often called character building. This is not true. It was awful. But it did make me determined to never repeat it again.

Least valuable experience

I'm afraid this is the point where I am allowed to rant. And it regards something which sadly is not confined to one year or even to medical school but will incessantly follow you through your career. It is called 'reflection'.

In the rush to modernise medical school and nurture 'continuous professional development' it has been decided that sitting down and writing a short 'reflective' essay about what you have just seen or done that day is the best way to learn and develop. I'm sorry, but I can honestly say that I don't believe this has ever helped develop my skills or knowledge as a doctor. It seems obvious to me that when something importance happens within your practice you will of course think about it and it will impact your future decision-making. This is called being a human being. But the problem comes when this becomes compressed into a set format and you are pressured to 'reflect' regardless of its appropriateness. It then becomes a box-ticking exercise, something that has to be done before Friday morning and something that is more of a hinderance than a help.

The future

And so to the future. One of the most abnormal aspects of medicine in comparison to other jobs is that from now until you become a consultant you continue to have a 'school year' structure. Unfortunately the three-month holidays during the summer come to an end when you graduate but none the less there remains a steady year-by-year progression throughout post-graduate training. Every August thousands of doctors from the most junior new graduates to more senior doctors in specialist training pack up their cars and move around the country to start a new job with a new title. From FY1 (new graduate) to ST7 (very senior registrar who is almost a consultant) there is a clear progression in seniority that has more in common with moving through school than it does with other professions. It is of course not quite that simple, and there are many hoops to jump through and challenges to meet including post-graduate exams and applications as well as the research and publications that you need in order to progress. Additionally though, there are fantastic opportunities to do things that are slightly different. Like many UK graduates my plan is to work in Australia following my foundation years and experience life in another, warmer, climate. There are numerous people that I know who have worked as doctors on treks in Asia and South America, who have worked in trauma centres in South Africa or emigrated to Australia and New Zealand. And although medicine can certainly be monotonous and infuriating at times, although it can be stressful and time-consuming and although you will go through moments when you regret your decision to choose it, it is this breadth of opportunity that presents itself post-graduation which, hopefully, makes it all worthwhile.

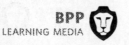

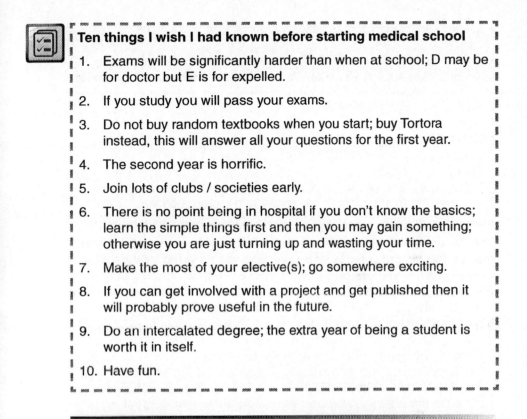

Ten things I wish I had known before starting medical school

1. Exams will be significantly harder than when at school; D may be for doctor but E is for expelled.

2. If you study you will pass your exams.

3. Do not buy random textbooks when you start; buy Tortora instead, this will answer all your questions for the first year.

4. The second year is horrific.

5. Join lots of clubs / societies early.

6. There is no point being in hospital if you don't know the basics; learn the simple things first and then you may gain something; otherwise you are just turning up and wasting your time.

7. Make the most of your elective(s); go somewhere exciting.

8. If you can get involved with a project and get published then it will probably prove useful in the future.

9. Do an intercalated degree; the extra year of being a student is worth it in itself.

10. Have fun.

Practical Guidance Tips

- The SL will sadly become an increasingly large part of your life as you progress and the exams start to pile up. However a lot of the time you spend there will revolve around chatting as opposed to studying so when it's time to get down to serious work it is not a bad idea to head up to the main library.

- Nobody ever died from a student trying to take blood or put in a cannula. So when you get the chance to try practical procedures you should get involved.

'But if you become a doctor, won't you be studying forever? ...and never get married? ...and have any babies?!'

Name: Sheetal Patel
Age: 23
University: Barts and the London
Course: Six-year MBBS, BSc
Year: Final
Extra info: Intercalated at KCL in my fifth year of medical school. First woman in my family to become a doctor

Year 3, Hillview Primary School, Malawi; parents evening: *'I'm afraid to tell you this sir, but your daughter will never achieve higher than a grade C in English, and that's only if she works extremely hard. To be honest, the same goes for all her subjects. She just seems to lack a certain insight..'* My father, a 30-year-old chemical engineer, never seemed to have heard such distressing words for his 7-year-old daughter. Of course, it was difficult to understand, *'your dad had a PhD in physics and chemistry, everyone else in the family is so bright, I don't understand what happened!'* That was usually the response he got when others learnt of my comprehension answers comprising mainly of *'because it says so in the passage'*. Sixteen years and a few more parent evenings later, he seems to be one of the proudest Indian dads I know, which is saying something! Remembering those words at 11.00pm, exactly two weeks into starting revision for finals and having done no revision at all, is definitely the prime time to share how medicine has been life changing for me.

How it all started

One fine evening in Malawi, a year and many many many hours of studying later, I made it, I came second in my class...from the bottom!' My joy of no longer being last was not exactly shared by my father. I guess I failed to see just how important education was to him. He worked insanely hard in an engineer shop in a small town called Limbe, just to put me through school. We lived in a poor one bedroom flat, where the bathroom was outdoors and occasionally infested with roaches, and weekly rubbish was dumped at the entrance. But despite the circumstances, spelling 'photosynthesis' was enough to break me out in a sweat! So yes, it was definitely a surprise when a week before submitting UCAS applications, I thought, 'why *not* medicine?'

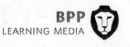

Medicine to me was initially status. In all honesty, it was a chance for me to prove to myself, and my family that I was capable of attaining a prestigious degree that anyone could be proud of. It turned out to mean a lot more than that. It meant being able to help others in a way that only a selected few could. To get to know their families sometimes even better than knowing my own, and to find that every skill you learn has a certain me-factor. I always felt I was an underachiever (surprisingly!), but it was the first time I took a bold step in making my own decision in what I wanted. I absolutely loathed doing repetitive and laborious work. Prescriptions, eye tests, dental checks, filing, accounts... it all drove me insane. Medicine promises flexibility, excitement but most importantly the room for development. My motivation was my past. I hated being told to live up to someone else's standards, to be like someone else, but most of all, what I can and cannot achieve. Although I did not see it all those years ago, my inspiration was my life in Africa.

Application

Deciding what to do was ok, but *where* to go? I must confess, for me it almost became a case of where will I get accepted? I studied Maths and Further Maths, which counted as a single A level, despite two very separate set of exams and grades! This restricted my options for universities. Finally settling on UCL, St George's, Barts and the London and Leicester, the blasted form was read, re-read and re-re-read before submission (although I still managed to spell 'opportunity' incorrectly, which will never happen again!). UCL was a university I looked up to. I felt the need to curtsey everytime I passed Euston! Clearly I focused far too much on perfecting my curtsey that I missed my BMAT, and was pleasantly rejected. *Opportunity* lost! St George's was a relatively specialised medical university with ethnic diversity (and a cousin), which in hindsight were probably poor reasons to apply, just as well, they required me to study a different subject to Further Maths when I was already half way through! Barts and the London, I fell in love with. Its traditional make up, ethnic diversity (it counts here!), HEMS, one of the top three research institutions in London, and the famous problem-based learning was hard to compete with. Leicester is my father's home town, and a place that I visited almost every summer after moving back from Malawi. The environment, people and a well-ranked medical university offering an MBChB provided sanctity from London, and became my sole 'outside-london' choice.

Applying was stressful. There isn't another term for it. It was most painful but definitely worth it. My first interview was at Leicester. I was petrified. Standing outside the interview door I felt like I was going to experience my first vasovagal syncope +/- jelly legs (not too sure about the medical term for this). The pressure to get a place was immense which was a perfect catalyst for working myself into a frenzy. Confusingly, seconds before walking into the interview room, it was clear; medicine *was* for me. Simply put, there was nothing else I would or wanted to do but this. It was probably the first time I truly believed it.

Times of sheer panic and doubt often set in during medical school, and I can only imagine it getting worse. But there is a reason why there are great doctors out there, and I am certain that a lot of it depends on the faith they have in themselves. Please note: not cockiness! So yes, after thinking to that depth in the time it took for me to walk to the interview room, I felt calmer. I was asked pretty standard and basic questions, '*Why medicine? What can you contribute to this university? What is our school known for? Where do you go when you come to Leiciester?* (?!)' Ten minutes and two weeks later, I got my first offer. As the only girl in my family to apply to medical school, a lot was at stake if I failed to get in first time. Taking a gap year would have meant battling against family and entering an alternative course. The relief was overwhelming. As corny as it may sound, that day in Hillview School turned from distressing words, to motivation, and finally achievement. Anyway! After all that, I didn't go to Leciester.

Barts and the London rejected my application. Although I already had a place, I wrote to them asking to justify why I did not qualify for an interview. Yes, it happens often and most the time, it's a waste of paper, but two weeks later, I was granted an interview. I'm still not sure how or why. I was asked completely different questions. '*How would you cope with death; predictable or preventable*?' Reasonable question. '*Being from a traditional background, how would you cope with marriage, kids and a job*?' My first thought after almost looking around the room to see if anyone else heard that was, '*You sound like my grandmother*!' But when asked whether I had a look around the campus, I almost lied. Fundamental rule; don't lie in interviews. After a brief shake of my head, the interview was over and I thought I screwed it up because my honesty may have been seen as a lack of interest in the university. Despite being content with Leicester University, I took a liking to Barts... lucky I got in!

Life as a final year medical student

So at the point of starting revision for possibly the biggest exams of my life, (I describe all exams like that including eye tests, but let's face it, these are slightly harder), a typical day starts out by attending a vascular surgical firm in Queen's Hospital in Romford – two hours from home. Leaving at 6.00am in the morning, fighting to get on the central line just to be squished by an elderly gentleman who now looks slightly happier, before finally making it in for a good grilling by

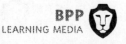

consultants. After hearing them suck in air through their teeth before grinning when you say you're two months from finals and don't know who pioneered vascular suture techniques, I scrub up for theatre to assist (it's a better term than retracting!). As ridiculous as it may sound, being this close to finals makes you feel like you need to know everything! I guess that's why it's funny seeing the panic set in the bleary eyes of fifth years. The afternoon is mainly taken up by clinics, examinations and presentations, after which I head home and attempt to study for a few hours before it's my favourite time of the day at midnight – bedtime.

At this point, there are still competency assessments in history taking, examinations, diagnosis, management and clinical skills, the only difference between third and fifth years is that now you *need to know* as a-soon-to-be doctor, compared to learning *just to merit pass* finals every year!

Assessments are important safety nets during training in medical school. If you miss learning a specific skill, it prompts you to complete it in order to progress to the next year. However I always felt they are more of a measure to teach us how to formulate our own assessments in preparation for when there are fewer checklists, and more blank subsections to complete before progressing up the hierarchy.

Social life

Admittedly I did not have much of a social life through the earlier years of medical school, but I feel that was due to poor time management and obsessive studying behaviour! But as the years progressed, I went out more. At the moment, logic dictates spending as much time as possible preparing for finals. However, my state of mind is much more stable when I set a 'target and reward' system. It allowed me to focus on chunks of revision in between going to see friends and family, and trying to fit in extra-curricular activities. This helped me more than studying for hours on end and never really focusing, either through lack of concentration or frustration due to retaining nothing and having even more to complete the following day. I realise now that if I carried on studying like that, I would have burnt out years ago. Don't get me wrong, you have to study hard and be sensible with the rewards!

Expectations versus reality

Starting at medical school is always starry. You dream that you'll be a great doctor, save lives, become a consultant and earn lots of money. It can happen, just at very different timeline in your head! I started medicine for all the wrong reasons, but am completing it for all the right reasons. The challenges medical school puts you through disciplines you second to none. Saying no to social events to prevent compromising revision, or pushing through the mockery on firms really thickens your skin no matter how sensitive you may be to begin with. It forces you to become a leader and a team player almost without realising – to bring forth different aspects of your own personality in a professional manner in order to engage with patients within minutes of meeting them; to become efficient with firms, time and resources; to learn how to control your temper, work well with colleagues and tackle your weaknesses. All in all, it's difficult to decipher when all this happens, but I can definitely vouch that it does. So you need to sweat and maybe bleed a little, but dare I say it's worth it especially if it can only get better and add to the initial dream.

What I love about medical school

I loved gaining the knowledge in order to understand and resolve a patient's problem. The feeling of getting something right and making someone better is indescribable. Although medicine is all very serious stuff at times, medical school always managed to make it light hearted; students and lecturers alike. Six years is a long time and so a bit of banter always helped!

The luxury of being able to spend your time doing what you wanted was brilliant, and a perk that I am sorely going to miss. The flexibility to waltz into whichever procedure I was interested in or, to stay with patients for longer than a clerking or a job or, to be with them through 15 hours of labour and welcome their baby boy/girl is unfortunately compromised once qualified.

I loved special selected study modules. They were essentially an opportunity(!) to learn about areas that are not necessarily on the curriculum. I learnt more anatomy, how to research and write articles, clinical studies and present interesting cases all in fields that interested me. It pushed me to overcome my fear of presenting and the extra work helped me confirm my interest and aspiration to pursue obstetrics and gynaecology as a future career choice. It also aided in making the choice to intercalate in a slightly more O&G (Obstetrics and Gynaecology) related BSc, which will hopefully help with future applications.

Above all, I have to admit, experience through my medical school has moulded me into who I am. I went from being shy, hypersensitive, unconfident and definitely not a leader, to being slightly less shy, sensitive, having a teeny bit more authority in what I say and able to take control of a situation. It may not sound like much but for me, it is plenty. The beauty about medicine is that it instills these qualities on top of being a safe and good doctor, as well as teasing out your weaknesses and strengthening them.

Being a student has its advantages – I hope to remember all the nasty things I have to endure as a student, whether it's ridicule, or no one appreciating the effort and time I put in to my work for them, either way, I'm going to try and avoid them when qualified.

For some reason, amnesia seems to set in with some doctors after 30 and they forget that they too felt like this at some point!

What I hate about medical school

Although I think assessments are useful, I *loathed* the paperwork (they tell me there is far more to come once qualified!). I couldn't stand remembering to haggle with doctors and other healthcare professionals to sign this and fill out that!

So you start with the expectation of learning 'cool medical stuff that will fix people', only to occasionally get ignored on ward rounds the one time you something interesting or valuable to say, because you're 'just a medical student.' I hate that term so much! I feel the need to make a public statement of never using the word 'just' and 'medical student' together. It is demeaning and somewhat insulting, especially when you spend hours sifting through notes and then no one wants to know the information they set you out on in the first place! (Ok, rant over – clearly that particular episode is still a little raw!).

Although the pressure of performing well in exams and impressing seniors grew every year and will continue to do so, at times it did become very difficult to deal with. There have been many many many times when I have stayed up to complete pieces of work and have a full day at the firm the following day, just to keep up a personal standard. There have also been times when having to say no to attend family weddings and holidays have been tough and occasionally have caused tears. The worst were exams. In my earlier years, I did not cope well and would literally have moments of giving up when I could not recall much of my revision despite hours of studying

...but these moments were also learning steps. They definitely make you stronger, more focused and determined not to miss events and to keep up with work. It is also comforting to know that high grade doctors also spill tears after a terrible day. The point is to learn to stay stable. Ironically, medical school helps with that too.

Most valuable experience

My vascular surgical rotation at Romford – this rotation is the most worthwhile. My consultant was traditional and old school. He regularly grilled me as with all my other rotations, but he also assessed me and took the time out to teach. He pulled me into his clinic and got me to see patients alone. He insisted that I do a full clerking, examination and present complete with no notes and hands behind my back. The man single handedly scared the living daylights out of me but really developed my skills to take a concise history, thorough examination and formulate a

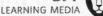

management plan. But he was meticulous as ever! One particular patient comes to mind. A middle aged gentleman with poorly controlled diabetes, smoker, over weight, hypertension, previous heart attack and notorious at keeping appointments. He had ulcers on his feet due to poor footwear. So come presenting time, I began with a background first. *Big* mistake. Everytime I spoke, he yelled out 'No!'. I tried to reason and again he yelled out 'No!'. Bearing in mind that the patient was in the room too, I felt myself match the colour of his erythematous skin! So that was followed by an actual three seconds of silence which is slightly short of an eternity to a surgeon. Eventually he laughed and said, 'I don't listen unless I hear the words 'presented with...'. It turns out that the patient had osteomyelitis and needed a toe amputation. Scrubbed for theatre and pondering about lunch, the consultant decided to teach me that hydrogen peroxide squirted into the now amputated toe in place of the ulcer helps kill anaerobes and looks rather like strawberry milkshake! I guess what I really learnt is that his old methods may not necessarily be perfect, but then again, old is gold.

Least valuable experience

Reflective writing. Year 1 reflecting writing was so painful, and I'm not talking about the 'painful but worth it' kind! It ate up a couple of hours every week and was absolutely pointless. We had to reflect on what a patient thought of our attempted history taking, after which it was reflected on again by the GP! Yes, I know this article is a type of reflection too, but this is different – I wanted to do this and it has a point! I don't remember anything from those exercises other than they really made my teeth grind!

The future

After writing this, I realise that so much has changed since I began medical school. I have high hopes for the future but have learnt that although I know the rough direction of where I want to be, I cannot plan it completely. There will always be changes. People that qualified a year ago and were determined to enter a specific specialty are now considering alternatives as their priorities in life change from perhaps career to family. Although I don't like uncertainty and risks, medicine is riddled with them. Risk and uncertainty arise every day and are perhaps the scariest aspects of the job. Our decisions as a doctor determine the outcome for the stranger who entrusted us with their most prized possession – their health. However, having said that, medicine also gives me the luxury to almost defy time. There is no age limit or strict pathways to follow. You can divert to whatever you get the opportunity to do should you want to. You can also leave medicine (which would be a terrible idea personally!) and have access to pretty much any job with your MBBS degree. Most of all, I love the unexpected. No day is the same as another in medicine. You are constantly

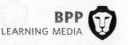

learning and discovering. How can that not excite anyone?! Unfortunately that also exposes you to some of the worst days of being a doctor.

I am concerned about not attaining an obstetrics and gynaecology post. I geared a lot of my selected study modules, elective and BSc towards it. Even worse, what if I change my mind and want to do something else? There is always that risk with medicine. I am most worried about making detrimental mistakes. The trust put into doctors is so great, it's better to not think about it at times to prevent rapid ageing and indecisiveness! However, here, ignorance is not bliss – it can be life threatening.

Moving away from such scary thoughts, I would love to take a six month research post in obstetrics and gynaecology in Australia. As a student I didn't travel much and I doubt I will be able to go away for as long as a couple of weeks at a time in the next couple of years, so here's to dreaming!

My family is obviously keen to get me married. But I don't think it is wrong to think that as a medic, you are three years behind the average course. We miss out on three years of personal development in the big bad world and this is always difficult to compromise on. That's not to say that it's not possible to get married or have a family during medical school, but that wasn't for me.

In hindsight, I have definitely made the right choice for me. Yes, I complain just like everyone else does, but I also love what I am doing and am excited by what I want to do in the future. I would advise budding medics to be sure that medicine is what they want to do. It is tough and will test you, but it is equally heartbreaking to learn that students start and then leave half way through because they do not enjoy it, or was not what they expected, but what I will say is important is to remain determined.

If my experiences have helped you even the slightest, then this reflective piece of writing will be the first to actually have made a difference.

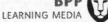

Ten things I wish I had known before starting medical school

1. As much as it is important that you get into medical school, make sure the university is also right for you – you'll be there for half a decade!

2. You will study so much, even trees in the winter will look like vascular arteries, and films like '*Abduction*' will make you think of the movement.

3. You will have doubts about entering the course – It's fact.

4. You will have to sustain embarrassment unfortunately!

5. It is competitive even once you've got in. If you're not a type A personality yourself, you will certain meet a few hundred of them!

6. There will always be something you do not know. Don't fight it – it's the harsh truth. (I still don't know who invented the suturing technique. Don't even know if it's a man or a woman!)

7. Don't use a gifted pen on your first day on wards, it will become a gift to someone else!

8. *Never* stand in front of a tracheostomy patient when examining their throat-you will get sprayed, or directly behind a patient when performing a per rectal examination for the same reason!

9. You do not have to be the smartest cookie in the group – you just need to be determined and work hard.

10. Learn to relax – you'll probably be exercising that skill the most!

Practical Guidance Tips

Guidance

- Although everyone is super keen to start off really well and learn everything there is in the mother book of Kumar and Clarke, they have been kind and given a concise version – a baby. Please use it, or the 'Cheese and Onion' (also known as the *Oxford Handbook of Clinical Medicine*). It literally has everything you need to know, but by all means, use the massive textbooks to reference and do some indepth reading from.

- There is already so much to learn, but try to conduct your own independent learning. You will do much better with minimal efforts!

- Remember that grades are not everything – everyone who qualifies will be a safe doctor. The competition starts afresh when you qualify!

Tips

- Stethoscope around the neck is a definite no-no, I'd say until you qualify!

- Find out how your consultant or registrar likes things done – whether it's presenting cases or reporting on investigations – you will earn happy points!

- Get involved. Some firms are great at involving students whereas, others are terrible. Either way, show you're keen and they'll definitely notice.

- Always unwind after a stressful day even if it is for half an hour before starting something else. It is vital to stay stable no matter how bad things get.

- Talk to others if you're feeling down. You'll be surprised as to how many students and doctors have felt what you might be experiencing.

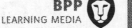

Chapter 6

The intercalating year: A dose of reality from five medical students

Lucy Robinson

Shahana Hussain

Jonathan Chun-Hei Cheung

Rathy Ramanathan

Fabienne Verrall

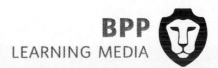

BPP
LEARNING MEDIA

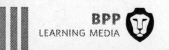

The intercalating year: A dose of reality from five medical students

'My intercalated year was probably one of the most valuable things I have done; partly because of the skills that I learned and partly because it proved to me just how much I really wanted to do Medicine.'

Name: Lucy Robinson
Age: 23
University: Cardiff University
Course: Five-year traditional integrated MBBCh
Year: 4
Extra info: Intercalated IBSc in Cellular and Molecular Pathology

I studied for my A levels at a small town comprehensive and was worried that this would put me at a disadvantage when applying for Medicine. However, through my hard work at A levels and my commitment to a vast number of extra-curricular activities I was able to secure a place to study medicine at Cardiff University.

My passion for science and desire to understand the intricate mechanisms underlying different disease processes drove me to complete an intercalated BSc course in Cellular and Molecular Pathology. I found intercalating a challenging yet very worthwhile experience. I learned about topics that interested me while gaining an appreciation of, and confidence in, a variety of academic and research skills (such as scientific writing, presentation and lab-work). I think my IBSc will definitely be of benefit to me in the future and will increase my employability.

I hope to share my experience of medical school and intercalation in particular so that future applicants can know a bit better what they need to expect!

How it all started

I first decided I wanted to do medicine after watching numerous episodes of '*Casualty*'(!). I was convinced that I wanted to be a paramedic as it would be a social job where I would get to help other people and also have the opportunity to drive a big, fast car!

However, various family members suggested that being a doctor might be a more suitable choice for my personality. I am very, very inquisitive and hate not knowing the answers to scientific questions. I am a practical person and

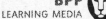

like to get things done. I appreciate the fact that as a doctor you get to play detective, solve problems and then work together as a team of specialists to find solutions. Also the fact that doctors get paid a lot was a nice bonus!

After reading a book as a teenager that included a character who suffered with diabetes I have always been fascinated by the condition – how it is a failure of one organ system that has so many ramifications for the rest of the body! It is a disease that theoretically should be completely treatable with insulin replacement therapy however it continues to challenge the medical profession in so many ways! It is a perfect example of the complexities of the human body and it is what inspires me to pursue my studies in medicine – I hope someday to specialise in Endocrinology and participate in the research for a cure for this increasingly common condition.

I assumed that this thirst for knowledge and determination to succeed would be more than enough to motivate me to get me through med school. I knew it would be tough but it was what I wanted to do so I was sure I would be able to manage the workload with a smile on my face and still have enough energy to go out partying till 2.00 am every morning!

Application

After my application I was convinced that due to my good grades and the amount of time I had spent involved in extra-curricular activities and conducting work experience in a variety of healthcare settings I was guaranteed to get four places at med school. Unfortunately things did not turn out to be quite that clear cut.

Months passed and I had not heard from any of my universities. This was particularly hard as many of my friends, who did not work nearly as hard as me and thus had much worse grades than me, received offers from all six of their universities! Eventually the time period for offers lapsed and UCAS recorded that I had been rejected from all of the med schools I had applied to. I was devastated. I had always maintained that if I did not get accepted first time round I would not apply again as it would be a sign that I was not good enough to succeed in medicine. My four rejections bought me crashing down to earth! I decided it might be best to climb down off my high horse and look for other ways to achieve my dream rather than giving up without a fight! I wrote to all four of the med schools asking if they could give me feedback on what I needed to improve to do better in the future. Cardiff were kind enough to write back and informed me that due to a computer error they had never received my application and they would be more than happy to give me an interview. As you can imagine this was a bit of a shock! I went for interview two days before the A level results were due. I was offered a conditional place and the

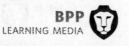

day I received my A level results and learnt that I would be attending Cardiff medical school ranks among one of the happiest days of my life!

Many people aren't so lucky. Many exceptional candidates miss out on places at med school every year just because of the sheer volume of applicants. It takes so many different qualities to make a good medic that the decision of who deserves a place and who doesn't must be an incredibly tough one! My advice to anyone who doesn't get a place first time would be don't give up! If you want it to, your medical career can last you a lifetime so a year out to reapply is nothing in the grand scheme of things. I am proof that persevering with med school applications is worth it!

Life as an intercalating medical student

Life as an intercalator is very different to life as a medical student. To start with there are a lot fewer lectures and a lot more time dedicated to 'self-directed learning'.

During an IBSc at Cardiff the year is split into two semesters during which time you have to complete 120 credits. The credits are usually made up of 7 × 10 credit modules and 1 × 50 credit research project. The modules cover a number of different topics: some are compulsory such as 'Research Methods' or 'Critical Analysis of the Literature' and some are optional such as 'Cancer Biology', 'Advanced Immunology' and 'Psychiatric Genetics'.

A typical day would normally comprise three to four hours of lectures followed by five to six hours of 'self-directed learning' time to be used for background reading, revision, in-course assignments and project work.

I chose to do a laboratory-based project as opposed to a library-based or clinical research project as I am considering pursuing scientific research or cultivating a specialist interest in histopathology as part of my future career. This meant I was expected to spend a minimum of two to three days a week in the lab. I assumed my time would be filled with pipetting, titrating, running assays and collecting data. In reality I actually spent a lot of my time reading about other people's work in the area, conducting calculations for and planning my own experiments, writing up my results and analysing data. I was lucky that my research was quite successful and that my supervisor was very supportive of my work but this also meant he was keen for me to spend extra time in the lab and often I ended up working late in to the evenings and at weekends.

Largely each module involved completing some form of coursework (ie an essay, a poster or a presentation) as well as a two to three hour end of module exam. The project required producing a ten-minute presentation and an 8,000 word dissertation. Having multiple assignments set at the same time was the aspect of the course that I found most difficult. As a medic, while the workload is heavy throughout the year, assessments tend to be scheduled one after the other allowing you to focus on each in turn.

The intercalated year was tough and I did have less free time than I would have liked. However it did force me to improve on my time management and I feel that the format of the year was probably a bit more reflective of what deadlines are going to be like during full time employment.

Social life

As a first year medic I would typically go out partying about two to three times a week. This included pubs, clubs and fresher socials (which would usually involve getting dressed up in ridiculous outfits and completing absurd tasks designed to make you drink more)! Nowadays I will still meet up with friends about two to three times a week but the activities involved are usually a little more sedate!

I would have liked to have been able to go out a bit more in first year if the workload hadn't been as much. I found it hard however adjusting to university life (cooking for myself and cleaning my own clothes etc) and my time management was probably not as good as it could have been.

During my intercalated year I did find myself more able to participate in extra-curricular activities but I think this was because I was better adapted to managing my workload and not in any way because it was an 'easy' year as many medics expect it to be!

Personally I find that societies that have regular meetings or training schedules are difficult to fit around the time and travel demands of the course. Many medics do manage it however and we are given Wednesday afternoons off to participate in sporting events.

Expectations versus reality

After achieving such good grades at school, I was convinced that while med school might be tough, I would easily manage the workload and a party filled social life at the same time! I assumed that despite the book learning most of my time would be spent helping treat patients and observing ER-like scenarios first hand.

The reality however was slightly different. I was shocked to find that I was no longer top of my class. I don't breeze through examinations like I used to and I often find myself turning down invitations to nights out just so I can stay in and study!

During the first two years of med school there was hardly any patient contact and instead my time was filled instead with lectures on protein structure and carbohydrate metabolism. The only time I have really been

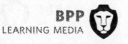

of any use to a patient was when I was instructed to hug a bag of saline to ensure its warmth prior to infusion. Not exactly the life and death sort of stuff I was expecting! But being able to help in that (very) small way was exceedingly gratifying and I am determined to keep studying because, as time goes on, I can feel my knowledge increasing and one day I hope to be a medic capable of directing such patient care.

What I love about medical school

In my opinion the best thing about doing medicine is the patients! I love getting the opportunity to spend time chatting to people about different aspects of their lives; Mrs Smith about her third grandchild's first steps and Mr Johnson about his tabby Bernard who refuses to eat anything but tuna fish from the tin!

Not only do patients end up sharing their most private thoughts and feelings with you but they also allow you to be present at very intimate moments in their lives. It is impossible to describe what a privilege it is to be so included; the look on someone's face when they are given the all clear from cancer, the sadness shared between family members as they receive bad news about an elderly relative or the joyful look on the face of first time parents at the birth of their long awaited child!

It is nice how the title of medical student often commands a certain degree of respect. When people are so grateful and gracious of what you are trying to achieve it makes the hard work seem all the more worthwhile!

Most of the time at med school I feel it is almost impossible to keep up with vast amounts of knowledge we are expected to know (and be able to recall at a moment's notice)! But there are certain 'light bulb' moments, where everything just seems to 'click'. There are the rare occasions when I can come up with an answer to a difficult question, identify an abnormality on an X-ray or can even name a possible diagnosis before I am told! I feel like these moments are increasing with each year of my training, especially after intercalating; as I am able to think in a more logical and analytical manner.

Med school is hard work. However everyone is in the same boat and this creates a great sense of camaraderie among med students! You face the trials and tribulations of placement together. You share conspiratorial glances with each other as you sit weary eyed seven cups of coffee into late night library study sesh and you celebrate together after you receive those all important pass marks.

What I hate about medical school

While a lot of the time it can be fun being surrounded by people who share the same interests and passions as you it can also get a bit tiring at times! I think certain types of people are driven to do medicine. Everyone at med school is a high achiever. Med students tend to be confident, opinionated and like to take charge. Sometimes it can be hard to stand out from the crowd and it is nice to have a group of non-medic friends with whom you can relax if the hectic world of medicine all gets a bit too much!

There is a heavy workload and it can seem never ending at times! It can feel like there are not enough hours in the day especially when you are given away placements that requires a lot of travel or difficult commutes.

Going to med school in Cardiff means you can be placed anywhere in Wales. The standard of accommodation varies between hospitals as does the potential for socialising with fellow medics. It can be incredibly isolating to be placed far away especially if you don't have the arrangements necessary to travel back to visit friends.

The medical course is a long one and with all the book learning and travelling around it can take a lot to stay on top and that is before you add in patient contact, never-ending clinics and multi-disciplinary meetings where you are expected to pay attention even though often you don't have a clue what is going on! The intercalated course is a mix-up of all of these issues combined with the stress of trying to complete a project involving original research. This is itself has its own issues; long hours, running the same experiments over and over again and a high risk that your research will fail through no fault of your own.

Most valuable experience

I found the first two years of med school, the 9 to 5 lectures and endless book learning, incredibly tough. At the end of the second year I wasn't even sure I wanted to continue with medicine! It wasn't till I started placement in the third year and got to see how the clinical process actually worked; a patient presents to a doctor, the doctor takes a history and conducts an examination, tests are run and ultimately a diagnosis and treatment plan is decided upon; that I realised that medicine is going to intrigue and interest me for the rest of life and is thus definitely worth pursuing. This sentiment was only confirmed by my year intercalating.

Originally I intercalated because I wanted to keep my options open, just in case I had decided against a career in medicine. Also, I have to admit, I am guilty of being one of those medics who assumed intercalation would be a nice easy year off in comparison to medicine! I found out the hard way that it definitely is not! Completing my IBSc in Cellular

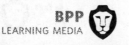

and Molecular Pathology allowed me to experience first hand the huge amount of scientific research that has to be completed in order to further our understanding even the tiniest bit! The experience was eye-opening and inspiring. I definitely hope to participate in other research projects in the future.

I would definitely say my intercalated year was probably one of the most valuable things I have done, partly because of the skills that I learned and partly because it proved to me just how much I do want to do medicine.

Least valuable experience

Some of the teaching during the first two years can seem a bit pointless to begin with! Clinically Cardiff schedules only five one-day placements in the first year of training and two one-week placements at the very end of the second year. These are supposed to enable students to acquire a taste of many different medical specialties but in reality the experiences are so short and spaced out that it is almost impossible to gain any real insight in to the working of hospital medicine at all!

The formal teaching (in particular pharmacology, radiology and analytical statistics) often goes too fast to grasp, especially when it can't be placed in any sort of clinical context! Whereas 'health in society' is dedicated such an inordinate amount of time it often feels that maybe the med school are trying to train you concurrently for Sociology degrees!

One-on-one tutorials are useful for consolidating all the aspects of your learning but often these can seem poorly organised and sometimes the tutors turn up so late it seems as if they think you have nothing better to do than wait around for them!

However I feel that none of the experiences you get at med school are entirely without value (so much so I chose to intercalate for another a year just so I could enjoy more of them)! As you progress through the later clinical years you begin to appreciate the logic behind why you have to spend so much of your first two years learning the basics before you can be let loose on patients!

The future

Before med school I always assumed I would end up wanting to specialise in Emergency Medicine. Emergency Medicine is the specialty you see most on TV and is often made out to be the most exciting specialty, where doctors work on the front line and save lives on a day-to-day basis. However as you progress through med school you realise it is not that glamorous and for every 'interesting' medical case you see there will be hundreds of other routine cases of alcohol intoxication and 'hurty-finger'(!).

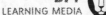

Luckily there are so many areas of medicine that you can specialise in! Endocrinology is my personal favourite – the multi-system involvement, the challenge of treating such varied diseases, the large amount of contact time between doctors and patients with chronic conditions and the potential for research in this every growing field! While I have considered specialising as a GP with an endocrine interest (because the hour and the pay is a lot better) my intercalated year has taught me that I enjoy learning about topics in depth rather than having a broad but general knowledge of disease conditions.

The current state of the NHS is a bit scary with the lack of finances and the constant administration rearrangements. I would love to work abroad when I am qualified and one of the attractive things about a career in medicine is that jobs seem fairly accessible almost all over the world (which might be useful to fall back on if work in this country becomes scarce)! Unfortunately the possibility of pay cuts for doctors in the future seems like an ever increasing certainty. When I originally applied to med school, I have to admit the promise of a good salary was an attractive prospect. However, med school is too hard to get through with money as your sole form of motivation. I was fortunate enough to find that my passion for medicine as a career has increased with every year of training (including my intercalated year)! While I have some regrets about not managing my time and social commitments more efficiently and the time, money and travel constraints of the course are great my desire to continue is strong. It is important you are sure of your reasons and dedication to medicine before you apply.

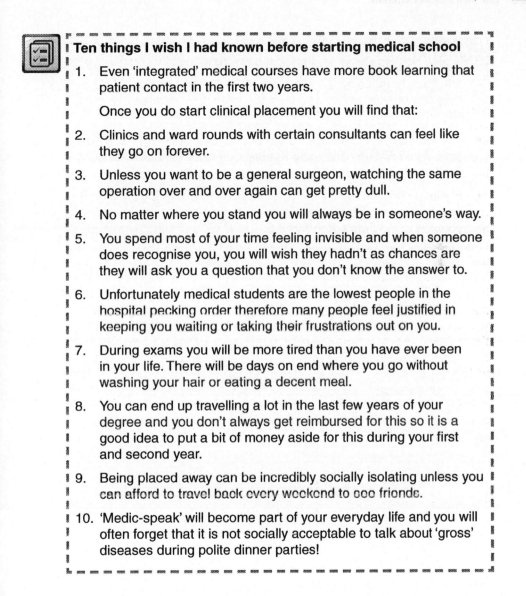

Ten things I wish I had known before starting medical school

1. Even 'integrated' medical courses have more book learning that patient contact in the first two years.

   Once you do start clinical placement you will find that:

2. Clinics and ward rounds with certain consultants can feel like they go on forever.

3. Unless you want to be a general surgeon, watching the same operation over and over again can get pretty dull.

4. No matter where you stand you will always be in someone's way.

5. You spend most of your time feeling invisible and when someone does recognise you, you will wish they hadn't as chances are they will ask you a question that you don't know the answer to.

6. Unfortunately medical students are the lowest people in the hospital pecking order therefore many people feel justified in keeping you waiting or taking their frustrations out on you.

7. During exams you will be more tired than you have ever been in your life. There will be days on end where you go without washing your hair or eating a decent meal.

8. You can end up travelling a lot in the last few years of your degree and you don't always get reimbursed for this so it is a good idea to put a bit of money aside for this during your first and second year.

9. Being placed away can be incredibly socially isolating unless you can afford to travel back every weekend to see friends.

10. 'Medic-speak' will become part of your everyday life and you will often forget that it is not socially acceptable to talk about 'gross' diseases during polite dinner parties!

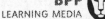

Practical Guidance Tips

- It is good to make an effort to hang out with non-medic friends as they can provide an escape from the everyday stresses of medic life!

- You can't expect to always be top of your class because at med school you will be competing against others as dedicated and hardworking as yourself.

- If you get the grades for med school you are obviously intelligent enough to succeed, try your best, and make sure you allow yourself some time out to relax.

> "Occasionem cognosce"; seize opportunity. This life is small but we
> can live on forever through the changes we make to other people's
> lives.'

Name: Shahana Hussain
Age: 22
University: Leicester University
Course: Five-year course
Year: 4
Extra info: Intercalating between third and fourth year of Medicine at
Leicester

My journey into medicine started after completing my A levels in
Mathematics, Chemistry, Biology, Philosophy and Critical Thinking.
Currently I am doing an intercalated BSc which involves a full year of
research and we are looking into assessing cardiac tissue damage and
the biological age of the heart post breast cancer radiotherapy. This will
then push back my graduation date to the summer of 2014 and then after
completing my foundation years I wish to pursue a career in Cardiology
or Paediatrics.

I have decided to share my own experiences because during my
application, I had researched a great deal about the application process
and course structures (including a discussion on a medical forum about
what constituted the *perfect* handshake) however I knew little about life
as a medical student.

How it all started

My decision to pursue medicine was highly influenced by my mother.
Having a parent who is a teacher comes with great advantages and
disadvantages; they will have taught students with a range of intellect so
when it comes to you – their expectations will be borderline impossible.
But on the other hand you understand the value of knowledge which
is of great importance in medicine as this will be your life's work; your
knowledge will be the vehicle you will use to change people's lives and
so *'ipsa scientia potestas est'* which translates as knowledge itself is
power and with great power comes great responsibility. This is the only
career in which you have the power to significantly enhance someone's
quality of life but wrongly used and the effect could be detrimental. To
prevent death – is there anything greater which you can offer humanity?

My decision was further reinforced during a placement with a cardiology
team. The consultant likened the process of diagnosis similar to that of

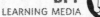

being a detective and methodically using the medical history and the relevant diagnostic tests at your disposal to pick up 'clues'. This is what makes medicine fun and almost seem like an art; no two patients will ever be the same so you must develop the art of deduction along with application of knowledge. However my expectations of medicine did not quite run parallel with the reality. Perhaps one of the most important lessons I learnt through my transition was 'common things occur commonly' – having an interest in rare disorders shows you are well read, however you should always utilise the Occams razor approach – assume the simplest solution first.

Application

I had an interest in research but also wanted to live close to home, therefore my first choice was Leicester medical school. The cardiovascular research group within Leicester is one of the best across the country and I would be able to commute daily. My second choice was St George's as they were also strongly research orientated, followed by KCL and Leeds.

My first interview was with St George's. On the day, I felt a mixture of nervousness and excitement; all these years of education, GCSEs, UKCAT, weeks agonising over the personal statement etc. was all for these 30 minutes of glory. These 30 minutes could then determine your entire career path and the lifelong friends you made.

The interview itself consisted of four interviewers; two final year students and two professors. The interview was quite challenging, with each interviewer asking four questions (not including questions following on from my answers). It ended with 'tell us the most interesting thing about you'. Unfortunately in the midst of revising for A levels, while also balancing volunteering with extra-curricular activities; one does not have much time left to be interesting. However looking back now, my fondest memory would be realising that the cow that Edward Jenner had obtained the cowpox from, was impaled on the wall of the clinical library. The next interview I received was from Leicester Medical School which was at the opposite end of the spectrum. There were only two interviewers and the interview itself was less of an interrogation and more a friendly conversation. There was greater focus on what makes a 'caring' doctor and patient centred clinical care. I felt much more confident in this interview. However as the interview only lasted 15 minutes I was sure I would face another rejection and began to plan a gap year if unsuccessful. Fortunately a month later, Leicester Medical School offered me a place and I was ecstatic to be accepted into my first choice.

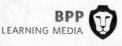

Life as an intercalating year medical student

Leicester Medical School has divided the five-year course into two phases. Phase 1 comprises five semesters; the medical school uses an integrated method of teaching so you get the best of both worlds; the traditional lecture based teaching followed by the PBL (problem-based learning) style of discussing clinical patient cases. Phase 2 is the clinical component of the course, it involves implementing the knowledge and clinical skills you developed during Phase 1, this takes place in hospitals and other clinical settings.

Assessments: The format of assessments varies from written exams to observed clinical examinations of patients (OSCEs), to writing a dissertation. The written exams are synoptic therefore each examination may contain material from the first day of medical school up to the day of the examination. During the third year of Medicine you sit the Phase 1 exam in January which consists of two written papers and an OSCE with 12 stations.

Typical day: During semester 5, you have three core modules as well as a student selected module and a weekly teaching session at a hospital, during which you are allocated to a clinician. The teaching sessions for the core modules are usually in the afternoons and last approximately four to five hours. This leaves the mornings free to complete the self study material in the workbooks or to undertake revision. For anatomy based modules you have a lecture in which you learn about the basic anatomy such as the hand, which is then followed by dissection in groups of the relevant anatomical part and then a tutorial session which involves discussion of the clinical aspects such as carpal tunnel syndrome. For the student selected module you can pick a scientific based module such as 'Vascular biology' or a language such as Spanish which depends on your preference but there is plenty of choice available.

There are approximately 20 hours of allocated teaching time per week during semester 5 and as a general rule of thumb I would spend an equal number of time self studying to the amount of teaching time therefore semester 5 required about 20 hours of self study and I then spent any free time revising for the Phase 1 exam – this would be approximately five hours a day.

Social life

Even though Medicine is a highly demanding course there is plenty of time to be involved in societies and to pursue personal interests. Many universities try to leave Wednesday afternoons free for all students to encourage participation in extra-curricular activities. Being a medical student encourages you to join societies more so because a doctor needs to be well rounded but also it's important to have a break from medicine

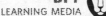

and develop other interests. For students reading this that are thinking about commuting – initially it may seem like a hindrance to having a social life but the converse is true – as you don't live within Leicester you tend to make more of an effort to get to know your fellow students (which is even more amenable with your own transport). During my first year, I was involved in organising a fashion show and also on the committee for the society 'Crossing Borders' as fundraiser, which aims to remove barriers to healthcare for refugees and asylum seekers, and was also involved in fencing. It's important to have a balance and good time management skills so you can get the most out of the university experience while also keeping on top of your work. I would advise getting involved in societies earlier on as in the clinical years later on – you will be on placements with demanding hours and planning your foundation programme application.

Expectations versus reality

The reality of life as a medical student greatly exceeded my expectations. For a start I had assumed there to be a great deal of competition amongst the students and I had read experiences of students at other universities even being told false information before examinations so that their fellow students could surpass them – however this is not the case at all in Leicester. All the students are willing to help each other; during each examination period there are numerous revision sessions being run by the older medical students for the years below.

What I love about medical school

There are a number of things that are great about Leicester medical school. The people at the medical school would be at the top of this list; the tutors are always willing to help if you have any concerns and the structure of the medical course is superb. Leicester has organised medicine in terms of body systems so for example when doing the gastrointestinal system we begin with the embryology then move onto the histology and anatomy, and follow through with physiology and pathology of the gastrointestinal system which is consolidated through group work sessions. Leicester is also one of the only medical schools in the UK which allow students to undertake whole body dissection on cadavers, from as early as the first year. The cadaver to medical student ratio is also quite small; 1:9 so you are able to fully appreciate the intricacies of the human body through explorative study. As mentioned earlier the course structure allows you learn in a structured environment while also gaining independence. There is also patient contact early on, you are required to write a dissertation at the end of Year 2 after having been following the journey of two patients through the 'People and disease' course for over a year. Each medical student is allocated two patients,

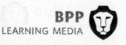

who both presented with the same presenting complaint but with two distinct disorders. This allows us to appreciate the importance of history taking as this will allow you to tailor a treatment plan to each patient while also gaining a 360° perspective into patient centred healthcare.

What I hate about medical school

There aren't many things I dislike about the medical school. However, being a daily commuter, the issue of parking spaces is my main concern. There is no on-campus parking available for students and a lack of parking space around the university becomes particularly problematic during morning seminars when you have to drive through the rush hour in the city and then search for a parking space nearby. Commuting is also expensive as fuel prices are rising regularly not to mention the many parking fines I have accumulated throughout the semesters. The best solution is to park in the student residential area which is a 15-minute walk from the university as it has free parking. But unfortunately driving for an hour and then having to walk is not the ideal way to begin lectures on a Monday morning.

Another dislike is on the topic of assessments – each paper contains 12 main questions topics such as a patient presenting with chest pain. These are then broken down into smaller sub-questions such as 'describe the histology of blood vessels' or the mechanism of a drug. Leicester does not mark papers in terms of overall percentage but you must pass each question individually so you cannot try to do well in one particular topic while avoiding another. You must have a good overall understanding of medicine, (which is beneficial when building up a good understanding of clinical knowledge and patients often present with multiple pathologies) but this can also be a hindrance as the exams are synoptic.

The medical school regularly provides feedback on performance in examinations, however this is in terms of which question topics you either failed or passed. No information is given on sub-questions or the total mark for that question. This was of particular worry during discussion with a fellow student on why pancreatitis can exhibit symptoms such as back pain. The student stated it was because the pancreatic enzymes begin to digest tissues and the back pain presents when the pancreatic enzymes digest the vertebrae. For this to be correct; the pancreatic enzymes would have to digest through the inferior vena cava before they could go further back and reach the vertebrae – and at this point the patient would have suffered fatal circulatory collapse before complaining of back pain. This is an example of why giving detailed feedback is of great value when it comes to healthcare.

Most valuable experience

Medical school isn't simply developing the knowledge and skills needed to treat patients; it is also about self discovery and changing your outlook as you progress throughout the course. The most valuable experience I gained was during Phase 2, while on my psychiatry attachment. I had always relied upon the 'biomedical model' as a framework when approaching the diagnosis to treatment cycle of a patient; where a patient's symptoms were directly a result of their underlying illness and management would include treating the underlying pathology. However through seeing many psychiatric patients I came to appreciate that the social and psychological state of the patient was also a heavy contributor to their illness as well as underlying biological abnormalities. I observed the treatment of a young woman who had an overdose for the fifth time and understood the impact of the emotional state on her physical health where treatment wasn't just curing her wounds but ensuring a healthy mental state so she would actively seek help during a relapse and to prevent further attempts of suicide, but to also ensure a healthy support network to aid her recovery back into the community. This approach applies to all disciplines of medicine and not just psychiatry.

Least valuable experience

My least valuable experience was during the first year; we all had to participate in a course called 'IPE' which stands for Interprofessional Education. This involved carrying out tasks with other members of the multidisciplinary team such as student speech and language therapists, nurses and occupational therapists. I appreciate the importance of these exercises as we will all be working as part of a multidisciplinary team to provide patient centred healthcare later on as clinicians in whichever specialty we decide to pursue therefore it is of great importance we develop those skills early on. However perhaps it would be better to implement such activities when we're further in the medical course such as during Phase 2 when we will have more of an experience of working within a multidisciplinary team. The tasks which we would undertake during an IPE session would vary a great deal, the one I was involved in was to produce an entrapment from a selection of materials such as paper, sellotape etc which would hold an egg. The task was then to drop the egg from a height of two metres and the successful multidisciplinary team would be the ones whose eggs didn't crack. Albeit a fun activity, one cannot relate the significance of it to a clinical scenario unless you liken the egg to the patient.

The future

Looking towards the future, I definitely want to work within the NHS as opposed to in a private sector however there are rising concerns

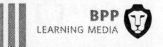

over the privatisation of the NHS gradually so predicting what the healthcare system will be like in 10 years' time is not an easy task. I have always had an interest in aerospace physiology and astronomy. The perfect job for me would be a medical officer aboard a space mission (well you should always aim for the stars as they say). However a more realistic career option is an academic paediatric cardiologist, this was an area I was interested in before medicine and I still wish to pursue this now in my fourth year. I would also love to travel and work with 'Doctors without borders' sometime in the future, where I can do the most good for the people that need healthcare so desperately. The great thing about medicine is that there a specialty for everyone; if you love excitement and working under pressure – Emergency Medicine. If you prefer an element of lab work and research – Academic Medicine.

In hindsight, I can genuinely say I have no regrets whatsoever about pursuing medicine. There will of course be difficult times throughout the course when you question whether this is the right career for you, and every medical student has considered this at one point however it will all be worth it knowing that you have made a difference to someone's life; however great or small that difference is. I hope that you have enjoyed my take on being a medical student and have got a small taste of life as a medical student. If you do not get in the first time; which is quite likely simply due to the high levels of competition for a small number of places then do not despair; try and try again. I would like to finish with 'occasionem cognosce'; seize opportunity. This life is small but we can live on forever through the changes we make to other people's lives.

Ten things I wish I had known before starting medical school

If I were to go back in time and see my younger self in the period before starting medical school there are some key pieces of advice I would give:

1. Do not buy any medical textbooks beforehand as the lecturers will advise on the most appropriate textbook for that and you can obtain copies from older years.

2. Do not to worry about getting to know people; everyone is in the same metaphorical boat. You'll make new friends in no time at all.

3. Achieving a less than outstanding result in examinations is not a major life crisis – you will need to adjust to being amongst an intelligent cohort of students.

4. Concentrate on your own learning and do not pay attention to what other students claim; those who claim that they haven't touched their textbook in the few weeks leading up to exams are usually those that revise profusely each night!

5. Enjoy yourself! Medical school will be one of the fondest memories you'll look back on and as it is a highly demanding course both intellectually and mentally, make sure you take full advantage of holidays.

6. It is okay to panic, each medical student goes through a period of being overwhelmed with work and thinking it's impossible to retain so much information but look around you – it's been done before and it can be done again.

7. You need to change the way you learn; simply because of the vast information you need to retain you will have to adapt your learning style and understand *why* something happens more than *what* happens.

8. People see you differently; you are now being seen as a professional and patients will reveal private aspects of their life to you. Appreciate the responsibility but also understand your limitations.

9. You will end up taking pro-plus to stay awake in the exam period and then nytol to fall asleep the month after. This is not a good idea.

10. Finally entering medicine was not the aim – that was just the beginning.

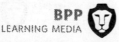

Practical Guidance Tips

- Before applying to Medicine, try to make yourself as much of a well rounded individual as possible. Make sure you have experience in most of the following five topics: music, language, travel, voluntary work and communication skills.

- Before your interview practise as much as you can! Practise in front of the mirror, practise with your friends, practise with mock interviewers. Don't memorise your answers as you will seem rehearsed and unnatural, instead make bullet points of things to mention.

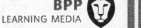

> 'Most medical students start their training with hope and
> excitement; but I started mine with despair.'

Name:	Jonathan Chun-Hei Cheung
Age:	22
University:	Newcastle University (MBBS); Imperial College London (BSc)
Course:	Five years
Year:	3
Extra info:	International student; have been a carer of an epileptic patient for years

My name is Jonathan and I am an international student from Hong Kong. I had been an engineering student before I entered medical school. I have already finished the two pre-clinical years at Newcastle University and am currently doing an intercalated degree in Surgery and Anaesthesia at Imperial College.

My brother has epilepsy. Therefore since I was small, I had to care for him. As you may expect, every time my brother had an epileptic seizure, people would look at us in a very annoyed way so that you could almost feel their gaze penetrating you. My brother was very lucky that he did not have any seizures following brain surgery a few years ago; but the impact of the disease has been debilitating.

I think that the readers of this book will most probably be secondary school students who are considering pursuing a medical career. So I want to make use of this opportunity to hopefully give you an insight into what the experience of medical school can be like for a carer of a chronic patient.

How it all started

I had thought about pursuing a career in medicine since I was in primary school quite naturally as my father is a surgeon and my brother is a chronic patient. However, there are several more practical reasons why I want to be a doctor. I will need a relatively high income-low risk job than an ordinary person would to afford the possible treatments my brother may need after my father, the only breadwinner in the family so far, retires. Having said that, I am fortunately interested in medicine. Being in a position that can help other families like mine is equally appealing.

Despite having chosen medicine, I did not (and still do not) have a high expectation of what being a doctor would be like. From the experience of taking care of my brother and seeing him trying different medications and being regularly seen by doctors, I have eventually learnt, although

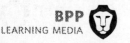

reluctantly, that the problems doctors cannot fix are in reality quite common. Even worse, there are too many things that we don't have a single clue about. For example, my father, an orthopaedic surgeon, has seen a lot of patients who are in pain. However, most of the time, it is just not possible to figure out the origin of the pain, let alone to treat it. Ironically, pain, albeit simple and common, is still something that we don't know enough about to treat effectively.

Being Chinese, I have seen many people considering seeing practitioners of Chinese medicine instead of those practicing western medicine. This is partly because of our culture; but in my opinion, this is plainly because of the paucity of our knowledge. I don't think Chinese medicine is worthless but I think it may work in a totally different way. Western medicine, on the other hand, is (said to be) scientific, yet what we know is too little and thus cannot stop patients from embracing the so-called 'alternative medicine'. These thoughts have made me cling more closely to patho-physiology than epidemiology, which I perceive to be similar to experience-based practice.

Application

I got admitted to the Medical Engineering course at the University of Hong Kong with my Hong Kong A level results (two Cs and three Ds) which, as you may expect, were not good enough to get into medical school. Therefore I planned to sit the GCE A levels and apply to UK medical schools during the first year of my engineering course. I didn't have the GCE grades before the UCAS deadline so I emailed literally every medical school in the UK asking if they would accept my results; I provided my HKCEE (GCSE equivalent in Hong Kong) grades, which included two Bs, few Cs and Ds for the total of eight subjects. I was absolutely stunned when I found that only fewer than 15 medical schools responded to my emails. Unsurprisingly, most of those schools said that my grades were not good enough, and the others asked me to refer to their webpage. So I only had to consider those schools which replied and did not turn down my application; these included Newcastle, Oxford, Cambridge, Glasgow, Bristol and Brighton. I excluded Cambridge and Bristol from my list because the others described their admission criteria in more detail. I also added Imperial's Biomedical Engineering to the five choices because you could only choose up to four medical courses.

During the application process, I was in email contact with several universities, mainly about the admission criteria, my exam scores, and interview details. Surprisingly, Oxford's admission office was the most willing to answer emails while Newcastle did not respond to my emails promptly.

The first email I received was from Oxford which informed me I was shortlisted for an interview. My referee and I then got asked by Glasgow and Brighton respectively about whether I could prove that I was able to achieve the predicted score (four As), which was not possible since I didn't have any new exam results then.

My experience gained at Oxford was very valuable. Applicants had to stay at one of its colleges for two days and had more than one interview. I got interviews in two colleges; one focused mainly on personality and the other on science knowledge, critical thinking and problem-solving.

The rejection from Oxford came 30 minutes after receiving the offer from Imperial. Receiving that rejection was quite frustrating. Alleviating the disappointment was the letter describing the reasons why I was rejected: my reference and exam results were not as good as others', so perhaps my performance during the interviews was not too bad.

A few months later, I got an email from Newcastle asking me to go to Malaysia for an interview. Compared to the interviews in Oxford, this one was more casual and there was only one interviewer instead of two. I managed to convince him that I could achieve the predicted score, which could be what got me the offer.

The story became simple afterwards – I fulfilled the offer's condition (3As at A level) and went to Newcastle.

Life as an intercalating medical student

The intercalated course I am undertaking this year has a different structure from that of a pre-clinical year. It consists of five modules. In the first three we simply have lectures revolving around various topics; in the last two most students would do a research project while I chose to take a specialist course on death, autopsy and law.

The workload so far has been very light. In terms of hours of lectures, this week we have 26. The rest is basically free time though you may need to spend one to two extra hours a week studying. Personally, I find this quite lenient because when I was studying Engineering, I needed to spend much more time keeping up with my course work. Moreover, this year in the intercalated course, about 40 or 50% of the course material has already been covered in the pre-clinical years.

Social life

I used to go to concerts with friends once or twice every month in Newcastle. After coming to London, I have gone to concerts less frequently purely because it costs more here. However, I actually have more free time now because of the reduced workload. This has been good news because I now can spend more time attending conferences and practicals like suturing workshops. This was something I couldn't do in Newcastle, partly because most events of this kind are held in London.

Many people think that medical students are always busy and therefore it is impossible to have a normal social life. This is actually not true. In fact, we potentially can have more time than others because medicine is generally easier than other science subjects and some students do spend more time enjoying themselves than others.

Expectations versus reality

Most medical students start their training with hope and excitement; but I started mine with despair because I was already aware of many limitations of the current medical field and of being a doctor. And no matter how hard I work or study I won't be able to eliminate the physical or social stigma that epilepsy has imposed upon my brother, or the many others like him.

Back to medical school – if you are hoping to see fierce competition in class, I am afraid you will be disappointed as there is nothing therein comparable to real competition. Very hardworking students and very intelligent students (the stereotypical image of a medical student?) are also rarely seen. At least I haven't known any yet.

Medical students, including myself, are not any smarter or more studious than other university students. In fact, passing the medical course, in my opinion, doesn't require high intelligence and diligence. The exams we had in Newcastle were multiple choice questions only, which were even easier than GCE A levels and required hardly any revision. This is all quite different from what I expected.

What I love about medical school

To me, the best thing about medical school is that you can be pretty sure that you can become a doctor after several years of education. Compared to students who study other subjects, medical students have a relatively clear career route; most of the time what they have to ponder is the choice of specialty but almost all of them are quite certain that they can become doctors. The extremely high employment rate is also very compelling. It is quite safe to say that all medical graduates will get a job within at most two years after graduation; at least 98% will get a job right away. This is far better than many other university graduates.

This is a particularly attractive factor to me because pragmatically speaking this feature is equivalent to being able to get a relatively high and stable income with a very low risk, which is what I wanted. And don't forget, you only need to get approximately 50% in order to pass. Furthermore, whether you pass with distinction, merit or just barely pass won't affect your qualification, although the chance of securing your ideal foundation job will partly depend on it.

Although the lenient assessments can mean that even if people do quite badly in the training they can finally become a doctor, I am glad that I don't have to undertake extra risks to accomplish my aim. After all, I want to be a doctor and being a medical student is merely a transition.

What I hate about medical school

I actually feel quite ambivalent about what I mentioned in the previous paragraph.

Strange as it may seem, medical school alone won't turn you into a good doctor. The whole process of application, interview, passing each year of the medical course until graduation doesn't truly screen for the best candidate to practise medicine. We all want our doctors to be competent, dedicated, passionate, empathetic, and hardworking. Sadly, however, graduating from medical school doesn't equate to the possession of any of these characters. This is one of the reasons why we can still see a lot of 'bad doctors' around.

Therefore, if one wants to become a doctor, he / she must be very clear whether he / she has the determination to pursue this lifelong career as the responsibility is not to be undertaken lightly; and once you enter medical school, passing assessments and proceeding to more advanced stages do not necessarily adequately equip you with the required skills. You must know very clearly what you need to do, what you want to do, and be motivated to do it. Just remember that it is very easy to be a mediocre doctor but becoming a doctor in whom patients can have faith is extremely difficult.

Most valuable experience

My most valuable experience was my two-day stay at Oxford because that was the first time I realised how easy it was to get into medical school in the UK – the required A level results were nothing more than a joke and the interviews were, albeit not simple, rather straightforward; and so that was the first time that I actually felt that I could achieve my goal.

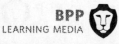

Least valuable experience

Some group projects are quite meaningless. Although medical schools often emphasise the importance of group work using the cliché that *'after becoming a doctor you'll have to work as part of the team'*, they usually don't think very carefully whether those projects can actually develop students' team-working skills and leadership. I am not trying to say that team spirit is not important; it is in fact a must-have attitude of a doctor. But the projects were just not ideal to foster these abilities.

The reason why a doctor must be able to work with other healthcare professionals is obvious: doctors on their own cannot possibly provide the healthcare that patients need. Yet the group projects often had a very low workload so that even one person was more than enough to do the task. Just like three-legged-running will never be quicker than running alone, trying to split a simple task into smaller tasks for each team member is simply ineffective, rendering the project futile.

The future

I will become not only a neurosurgeon but one that patients can have faith in. I hope every patient, especially those whose disease was not due to their fault, like intellectual disability, will be treated seriously and with respect. Mentally disabled patients are often put in a position of disadvantage. If even some doctors, who should treat all their patients equally, treat them with a dismissive manner, then whom can these patients seek help from?

Even if I am not able to change this culture, I would be able to at least provide some help. It's true that there isn't any treatment that can directly improve their quality of life, but there is still something that a doctor can do to support them, such as keeping detailed medical records and offering them appropriate medical certificates.

Ten things I wish I had known before starting medical school

Nothing. So far none of my experience in medical school has changed my decision. Although not everything I expected was exactly true, I have never regretted the choice I made.

Practical Guidance Tips

- Choose a specialty before you apply.

  Although it is kind of obvious and perhaps controversial, you should definitely choose a specialty before you apply. The reasons behind this are quite simple.

  - Not having a predilection can mean less determination and less knowledge as to what a doctor is like. If you were a patient, would you choose a cardiothoracic surgeon who decided to be one even before entering medical school or one who chose the specialty just because he / she happened to get into the field?

  - You need to start preparing your CV as early as possible. Otherwise it's quite difficult to contend for a place in the more competitive specialties like neurosurgery.

- Always remember to put yourself in the patient's shoes.

  Medical students are often passionate and empathetic when they first enter medical school. But as they progress, these characteristics tend to burn out. This can be ascribed to how we are trained – although the importance of empathy is stressed in our education, keeping somewhat emotionally isolated from patients is much less distressing.

  Nevertheless, this is not an excuse for not trying to understand the predicament that the patient is experiencing.

> 'Medical school is a unique experience and an amazing opportunity, make the most out of it!'

Name: Rathy Ramanathan
Age: 23
University: University of Liverpool
Course: Five years with an additional optional one-year intercalation
Year: 5
Extra info: Intercalating BSc – Imperial College, London

I came to university straight after completing my A levels at the age of 18. I have now completed four out of five years studying medicine at the University of Liverpool, and am currently taking a year out of Medicine to study an intercalated BSc in Medical Sciences with Endocrinology at Imperial College, London.

Getting a place at medical school is becoming extremely competitive and surviving at medical school can be difficult at times. I have therefore decided to share my experiences of applying to study medicine and what life is really like as a medical student. I think it is vital to learn about peoples' experiences in order to know what options are available, and to know the true facts about whether this profession is suited for you.

How it all started

My first thoughts in pursuing a career in medicine were inspired by viewing my cousin's constant struggle for life due to a mitochondrial disorder. Visiting the intensive care unit in hospital on a regular basis allowed me to observe the multidisciplinary teamwork of all the healthcare professionals, strenuously working to provide all aspects of patient care. This extremely impressed me, and was my principle motivation to study medicine. My work placements, carried out in the Accident and Emergency and Gastrointestinal departments, were fascinating experiences which reinforced my decision to commit myself to study medicine. I loved the buzz and excitement of the Accident and Emergency department and not knowing what patients with varying severities would present. Further, I was thoroughly impressed with the latest advances in medical technologies of using a flexible tube with a camera and multiple gadgets on the end of it to investigate, diagnose and treat patients in the Endoscopy department.

Having been exposed to many medical situations and from speaking with doctors, I knew a career in medicine was not to be taken lightly.

I realised a lot of commitment was required to study for five years as well as Medicine being a demanding and continually challenging course. A well known phrase I had heard being used to describe medical students is that they work hard and play even harder, so I thought at the time, at least I'll be able to enjoy myself after all that hard work!

Application

I went to many university open days across the county and finally selected to apply to St George's University of London, Barts and The London School of Medicine and Dentistry, University of Liverpool and University of Glasgow.

I applied to St George's and Barts due to their location. London is a vibrant city, there is always something happening and it is extremely diverse which is why I applied there. Having lived in Scotland, I thought it would be a good opportunity to go back and experience again the places I love in Scotland, which is why I applied to study at Glasgow University. My final place I applied was Liverpool University, because I had attended the open day and I was thoroughly impressed by the available opportunities and resources as well by how friendly the people were.

Applying to medical school has been the most stressful time in my life. When you want something so badly, every part of the application needs to be done to perfection in addition to keeping up with your A level studies to achieve the best grades possible. I had many sleepless nights worrying and stressing over what would happen and if the dream would actually become a reality.

The interview process was the next hurdle to jump through. I was thrilled to get interviews initially however the actual process was daunting. I had many concerns, what if they ask me something I don't know anything about, what if I say the wrong thing, what if I don't show them how much I really want this and why I really do deserve a place etc? Looking back the questions were not too bad. Most of the people on the interview panel were friendly and actually wanted you to do well.

Checking on the UCAS website after my interview and finding out I had got a place, I was ecstatic. Words can't describe how happy I was that day. While being so happy, I realised I now needed to ensure I met the conditions of my offer and worked as hard as possible for me to get the best grades I could possibly achieve.

The application process is tough. Some form of selection process is required though by medical schools as so many students are achieving the best grades and it is extremely difficult to decide which students are the most suitable for the limited number of places at medical school.

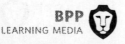

Applying for my intercalated BSc was a totally different experience. It was a lot less stressful compared to applying for medicine. Some medical courses are a six-year degree eg Imperial College London, University College London etc, so you will study medicine for five years and at some point in the course spend a year doing a BSc, and therefore you will not be required to apply specifically for the BSc course. Most other universities make it optional to do a BSc and again it varies between universities when during your medical degree you do the BSc. All universities allow you to intercalate either at your home university in a different department or at another university. An application form is required to be completed when applying for intercalated degrees about six to nine months before the start of the degree. Different information is required depending on where you apply and the course you apply for, so exact details and deadlines for submitting applications need to be referred to the relevant university websites.

Life as a intercalating medical student

As an intercalating BSc student I am back to being taught in a lecture theatre with no clinical contact. My typical day involves around 13 hours of lectures a week with a few hours of tutorials per module. As this course is a BSc there is a lot more free time and you can feel like a normal university student compared to your medicine timetable where you start to feel like an unpaid doctor! There is approximately one and half free days per week. Another good thing about the BSc course compared to medicine is that Wednesday afternoons are always free and so you can commit and get involved with university clubs and societies.

As with any intercalated BSc course, the teaching is very much focused at a molecular level with references to its clinical application. My course aims to teach the forefront of endocrine research and therefore requires students to read lots and lots of articles. The workload is manageable; lecture notes and reading lists are available, as well as lecturers being willing to arrange tutorials on difficult topics which is helpful. Roughly one to two hours a night is required to read through the lectures and ensure you understand what has been taught. My BSc course is split into three parts, the first part is a two-week introduction to the BSc course, the second part is three five-week taught modules and the final part is a ten-week module. After completing the BSc introduction course which refreshes your knowledge of the skills required in your BSc year and the three five-week modules, the final BSc written assessments are in February. The exams are very different to medical school exams where we are used to answering single best answers and multiple choice questions. As these are BSc exams they involve answering short answers, short essays and long essays; a skill I have not used since my A levels! I am required to submit two pieces of in course assessment every module which include critically appraising articles and writing essays. I then have a ten-week module to carry out a research project for which I need to submit a 5,000 word report and undergo a viva. There is also the option of doing a five week taught course in history of medicine, medical humanities or death, autopsy and law, followed by a five week mini project instead of doing the ten-weeks research project. Even though the assessments are very early in the year, they allow you to get it over and done with so you can then completely focus on the BSc project.

Social life

As an intercalated student, there is a lot more free time available compared to when you are studying medicine. I am involved in many societies; I am the joint co-ordinator of a society that teaches basic life support to school aged children, and the treasurer of Marrow, a society that recruits people on to the bone marrow register. I am an active member of the International Tamil Society and Hindu Society. There are also a few other societies eg Medsin, Cooking Society etc which I cannot commit to on a regular basis but I wanted to get involved and so attend whenever I'm free. I would recommend to make the most of the intercalated year and get involved in as many societies as you want to as it is difficult to do them all when you are on clinical attachments. Time management is an extremely important skill as a medical student and doctor. You need to take time out from the course to do the things you enjoy otherwise you will start to feel insane. The key thing is managing it all into the time available and making sure you have fun but are keeping on top of your work as well. Extra-curricular involvement is vital, all students need a break from medicine and taking part in societies provide the perfect opportunity to do things you enjoy and won't otherwise get the chance to do. It also gives you a chance to make new friends as well as improve your CV.

Expectations versus reality

It may be daunting at the start being a medical student not knowing what you are expected to know. The reality is that every doctor has been in your place before as a student, and understands it is a very steep learning curve. As long as you are enthusiastic and willing to learn, most doctors will help and support you.

When starting at university, studying medicine for five years sounded like a long time, and so even contemplating studying another year to intercalate seemed bizarre! But your time at medical school really does fly by and so spending another year as a student actually does sound appealing!

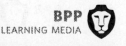

What I love about medical school

Medical school is one of the best times in your life and will allow you to grow as a person. What I love about medical school is the opportunities it provides. Medical school is a close kit community as you are there for long time, and your fellow peers become your close friends and are pretty much like your family! Everyone is in the same boat and able to share the experiences of your best and worst times together. Medical school provides a safe environment in which to learn medicine, make mistakes and to learn from them for the future. Participating in the multidisciplinary team, getting hands on experience and patient contact during clinical attachments is the best part of the medical school. Doctors are very busy and are only able to spend a limited time with patients. This is totally different for students; we can spend as long as we like talking to patients, understanding the impact of their disease on their lives and sometimes are able to acknowledge and address their concerns. Even as a student, you can make a difference to peoples' lives.

What I hate about medical school

Medical school provides challenges which may sometimes start to feel overwhelming. Medical school is a place where you will be challenged to study a vast volume of information and you'll retain more knowledge than you ever thought possible. It is vital to study as you are going along through the year as it is easier to learn concepts closer to the exams that you already understand. Not everyone learns in the same way though, and some people do prefer working the bare minimum during the year and then a month before exams spending many sleepless nights in the library cramming all the information, while maxed out on caffeine!

Another thing about medical school is that they are training you for a career in medicine from the first day you start. This means you will always find you have the most lectures, timetabled teaching, attachments and the least amount of holidays compared to other university courses. Therefore, I recommend you make the most of any holidays given as they don't come often.

Competition does occur between students in medical school. I personally suggest competing against yourself to do better and achieve the best possible marks. There is no point worrying and stressing what other people are doing or how much other people know.

Most valuable experience

The most valuable experience during medical school was the opportunity to do a research project during my intercalated year. Doing a research project allowed me to do either a scientific or clinical research project

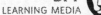

and to learn the relevant skills required, which you otherwise would not get a chance to experience during your medical school training. Doing a project allows you to address questions at the forefront of medical research which is an exciting prospect. This then will give you the opportunity to present your work at conferences, win prizes and to get publications, all which are added bonuses for your CV.

Least valuable experience

The least valuable experience during medical school was having a log-book to complete during clinical attachments. When having a log-book, students become very focused on completing everything that needs to be signed off in order to successfully complete the rotation. This limits the learning experience for students as they become uninterested in seeing cases and doing procedures not included in the log-book, and therefore not fully participating in the team during their clinical attachment. Students need to be reminded that regardless of the log-book, one day they will be a doctor and hence it is crucial to witness as many experiences as possible during clinical attachments at medical school.

The future

In the future, I'm still not exactly sure what I want to specialise in. I've always known, even before starting medical school that surgery wasn't for me. I am currently considering a career in endocrinology, paediatrics or general practice. Having done my elective, clinical attachments and from my personal experiences from working with children, I believe a career in paediatrics would be suited to me. On the other hand, I am currently doing my intercalation year as well as having done several special study modules and audits in endocrinology and am deeply fascinated by this area of medicine. General practice is also another rotation I have always enjoyed on placement. I am particularly drawn to this field due to the diversity of patients and the continuity of patient care which is unique to general practice. Nevertheless, I still have time even as a junior doctor to decide for definite what I want to do in my career. What I love about a career in medicine, is the patient contact, problem-solving challenges, the fact it is a very rewarding career and you can make a difference to people. However with any career, there are some drawbacks to a career in medicine, it is very competitive to get jobs and you are required to work long hours in order to gain the necessary experience. My career aspirations are to do some medical research however to mainly have a clinical role as this is was interests me the most. I currently don't know what specialty I'll be doing in 10 years' time; but as long as I'm happy, able to work and making a difference to people, I will be satisfied!

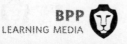

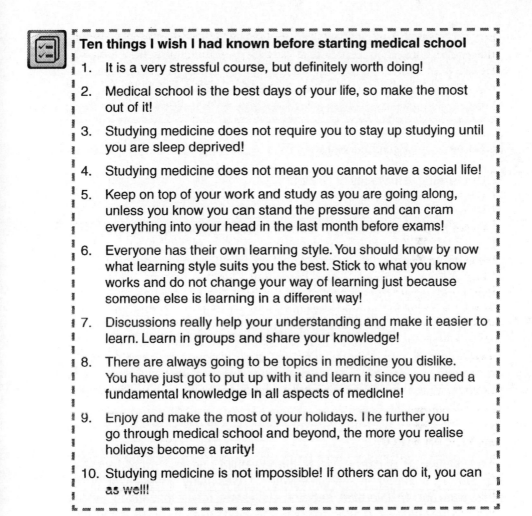

Ten things I wish I had known before starting medical school

1. It is a very stressful course, but definitely worth doing!

2. Medical school is the best days of your life, so make the most out of it!

3. Studying medicine does not require you to stay up studying until you are sleep deprived!

4. Studying medicine does not mean you cannot have a social life!

5. Keep on top of your work and study as you are going along, unless you know you can stand the pressure and can cram everything into your head in the last month before exams!

6. Everyone has their own learning style. You should know by now what learning style suits you the best. Stick to what you know works and do not change your way of learning just because someone else is learning in a different way!

7. Discussions really help your understanding and make it easier to learn. Learn in groups and share your knowledge!

8. There are always going to be topics in medicine you dislike. You have just got to put up with it and learn it since you need a fundamental knowledge In all aspects of medicine!

9. Enjoy and make the most of your holidays. The further you go through medical school and beyond, the more you realise holidays become a rarity!

10. Studying medicine is not impossible! If others can do it, you can as well!

Practical Guidance Tips

- Enjoy your time at medical school and make the most of every opportunity.

- Time management is essential to do well in medical school and also have an amazing experience.

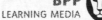

> 'Sometimes medical school feels like stepping into a different world, with its own language, culture and clothing. It may sound daunting, but there is an immense sense of unity and camaraderie, which makes you feel like you belong.'

Name: Fabienne Verrall
Age: 21
University: University of Bristol
Course: Five years
Year: 3
Extra info: Intercalating in Bioethics BSc – third year of study

I was about 7 years old when I set my heart on becoming a doctor. Cliché, I know! Funnily enough, I also knew that I wanted to come to Bristol. I didn't understand the concept of university at 7, but I kept hearing 'Bristol' and 'University' in the same sentence and it sounded pretty good, so I decided to keep that in mind for 11 years' time. I later found out that my older cousin went there, so that explained a lot. I went to a really good mixed catholic comprehensive school and college, where the support I received was fantastic. I studied the standard medical trio of A levels: Biology, Maths and Chemistry, but I mixed it up with a bit of Philosophy and Ethics.

How it all started

As I confessed earlier, I was a strange child and knew that I wanted to pursue a career in medicine when I was fairly young. Obviously, this was not an informed decision as I was really influenced by my grandfather being a doctor. He was the kindest man in the world and my role model for many years. As I grew up and began to understand what a career in medicine would entail, it sounded more and more attractive. I wanted my career to be vocational and immerse me into a professional community, one which allowed me to work with people who are vulnerable and are in need of care, as well as a career that would allow me to become an expert in a particular field.

My expectations of medical school were surprisingly accurate. I expected it to be intense, exhausting and exciting. Above all, no matter how hard it gets, I believe that it will all be worthwhile in the end and from my experience so far, it lives up to all my expectations.

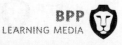

Application

If I could go through the application process again, I would do it very differently! I wouldn't have wanted the outcome to be different, as I love Bristol. But if I'm brutally honest, I think I picked universities for the wrong reasons. I applied to Southampton, Bristol, King's College and the University of East Anglia. When I reflected upon the universities that I had chosen, I realised they were all about two to three hours away from my home. Subconsciously, I think I was making sure that I wouldn't be too far away. I'm not saying that you shouldn't take location into account, because it is definitely important, but it shouldn't be the deciding factor. Just don't let it stop you looking at fantastic universities that are further afield. For example, Edinburgh is an amazing university and I didn't even consider it because it was hours away.

During the application period, I was stressed! I was the only prospective medical student in my college, so the teachers constantly asked me whether I had received any letters / emails. It was nice that they cared, but as the months slipped away, their expressions began to worry me. It got to April and I was beginning to consider planning a gap year, when I was invited to an interview at Bristol. I can't tell you how relieved I was! The following week, King's College offered me an interview, so a little bit of faith was restored. The day of my Bristol interview was a blur. I was the definition of nervous. I stepped into my interview and my nerves strangled my vocal cords and nothing came out. The first question I was asked was what I enjoyed the most about my study of ethics. I had anticipated this question as it was smack bang at the top of my personal statement and the study of ethics is paramount in medicine. I had all the knowledge, but my mouth wasn't connected to my brain at this point. I had to excuse myself for a moment, collect my thoughts and give myself a kick up the backside! I stopped thinking about the importance of the interview and told myself that this was just an opportunity to talk to medical professionals about my work experience. As soon as I changed my outlook on the meeting, the words flowed and there was a glimmer of hope.

A week later, I received a letter from Bristol saying that they were delighted to offer me a place and I was over the moon! My interview at King's College was the following week and was much better than my Bristol interview, but I didn't get an offer. I think I was too relaxed after receiving my offer from Bristol and maybe the interviewers sensed my lack of enthusiasm.

Life as an intercalating medical student

I'm currently intercalating in a BSc in Bioethics. This is divided into three subjects which are medical law, bioethics and philosophy. On average I have six to eight hours of contact time a week, which is made up of one to two lectures, three to four seminars and a fortnightly law tutorial. This is a dramatic change from last year when I had lectures from 9.00am-5.00pm most days.

A typical day in the life of a Bioethics student would go something like this:

9.30am – 11.30am: a lecture on ethical theory eg Deontology

1.00pm – 2.00pm: a research seminar eg Compromise between Law and Ethics

2.30pm – 4.00pm: a medical law seminar eg The Importance of Confidentiality

That's considered a very busy day! We would definitely need to go to the pub after that! It's really hard to quantify my free time, as I do my pre-reading and assignments sporadically during the week, so I don't really keep track of when I'm 'free'. I also have a part time job for 12 – 14 hours a week, which possibly indicates how much 'free' time I get.

In the second year we received a few presentations on the benefits of intercalating. So many people wanted to intercalate because they thought they could have a 'doss' year. It is far from a doss! It is a completely different way of learning, as it is very self- directed. Bioethics is assessed primarily on a 15,000-word dissertation, a 5,000-word ethics essay, three 2,500-word law essays, a three-hour philosophy exam and a few more formative essays and presentations. So basically it's a lot of reading and a lot of essay writing, which is really difficult when you've just studied science for the last few years. It has really highlighted just how 'spoon fed' we are as medical students. We are given large amounts of information to simply digest and move on. In humanities, the concepts require much more thought and reflection. We have studied several topics which have gone right over my head! That never happened in Medicine. So my advice regarding intercalation is to make sure you really enjoy the subject, because you need to be motivated as it involves lots of hard work! If you enjoy the work, it is really fun and gives you an extra year as a student, before hospitals become your new home!

Social life

Due to having more free time, I feel like I can be a proper student this year. By proper student, I mean having lie-ins, going to lectures at 11.00am instead of 9.00am and trying out some strange hobbies! I go out about three or four times a week which is definitely starting to catch up with me. I'm the captain of the Medics Women's Football Club, I'm involved in the Obstetrics and Gynaecology Society and I go to a Cuban fitness class. I also joined the Food Society and the Chocolate Society – best decisions I've ever made! Most medics do extra-

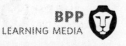

curricular activities and I think one reason is because it is escapism from the intensity of the course. I do it to keep fit, to relax and to have fun. It is also another way of making friends and it's a laugh / delicious.

Medical students love going out! I know lots of people in my year that went out just as much as any other student. Whether they did any work is another matter entirely! In all seriousness, if you can manage your time well, then you can be free to do whatever you like. You just need to keep on top of your work and know your limits. Don't get too tired and run down, as the workload will get the better of you. Then the lunchtime drinking and excessive ice cream consumption begins and it's a slippery slope from thereon in.

Expectations versus reality

My expectations of medical school were centred on the notion that it was going to be difficult and therefore I was going to be miserable for a few years! I think I got this idea from observing doctors, realising how much responsibility they had and comparing that to how little I knew. The equation didn't make sense! How do you go from my position to theirs in just five years? I think the answer is that it takes five years to understand the basic principles of being a doctor but years of practise to understand the profession. Lecturers at medical school don't expect you to be perfect straight away, but they expect you to be enthusiastic. I'm glad to say that the reality of being a medical student is fantastic. Whenever I think I'm miserable, I'm nearly always just a little hung-over. Watch out for that one.

What I love about medical school

One of the things that I love most about medical school is the sense of community. The year groups are normally between 200 and 250 people, which means that lots of people are in the same boat as you. The course is challenging and sometimes intense, which I think brings people closer together because you experience everything at the same time. Sometimes medical school feels like stepping into a different world, with its own language, culture and clothing. It may sound daunting, but there is an immense sense of unity and camaraderie, which makes you feel like you belong.

Another aspect of medical school which I love is how it attracts particular characters, so you meet very like-minded people.

Medics are renowned for going out and enjoying themselves and from experience I would agree with this reputation. We have amazing socials, which cause the worst hangovers known to mankind, but are riddled with gossip and are talked about for ages.

As I mentioned earlier, medics love their extra-curricular activities and I have really enjoyed being part of the societies and sports clubs. In the first year, I remember walking out of Medics' Freshers' Fair with a bunch of leaflets about the dozens of different societies, sports teams and charities you could belong to within the medical community. I was overwhelmed!

The experiences don't stop there either. Being a medical student provides you with limitless opportunities in education, research, fundraising and travelling. If you are really passionate about a cause or a topic within the scope of healthcare, there will be someone who will support you. There are so many chances to do really rewarding work, before you've even qualified.

Ok now I'm going to sound really nerdy. The reason I know that Medicine is the right course for me is because I enjoy studying lots of different subjects. In the first two years we studied biochemistry, anatomy, pharmacology, physiology, sociology, psychology, law and ethics. There were also opportunities to study languages, philosophy, art etc. There aren't many courses that dip into everything! Now I'm studying law, ethics and philosophy in much more detail and I think it's a privilege.

What I hate about medical school

The flip side of meeting like-minded people is that they tend to have similar character traits, for example – competitiveness! The course may be hard, but everyone is really clever. That may seem obvious, but you will meet people who are beyond the realms of what was deemed clever at your school. I hate how people are always desperate to find out everyone's exam results and how some people are reluctant when you ask them for help! My advice would be to stay away from these people during exam periods and focus on your own goals.

The workload is not something that I hate, but I don't enjoy the resulting implications. For example, Christmas and Easter holidays should be renamed 'study leave', because this is essentially what they are. Medicine has more exams than most subjects, so you need to get used to revising. I used to get annoyed when my non-medic friends were going Christmas shopping together while I was stuck at home with my head in a book. It's not that I was being naive about what the course entailed, but the reality stings sometimes. Of course you have to balance revising with having breaks, but every time I went out I felt guilty.

Something that I find myself doing frequently is thinking about the future and I think a career in medicine encourages this. You're bombarded with information about different specialties early on in medical school and forced to think about what you might want to do. There is absolutely nothing wrong with this, but it definitely makes you think about the next five, ten, fifteen years. You'll have friends on other courses who won't know what they're doing tomorrow, but you may know how you want to spend the next twenty years and they'll probably be defined by your career.

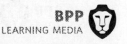

Some people may have this aspect in their 'love' section, but it annoys me sometimes as I feel like I'm living in the future rather than the present.

Most valuable experience

My most valuable experience so far, would have to be an exercise that we did in second year called 'Consultation Skills'. We were given a small amount of teaching at the beginning of each session and given a scenario that we would have to act out with an actor taking the patient's role. The actors were fantastic, which made the scenarios scarily realistic. There were some truly tragic scenarios and the reality is that in a few years – these won't just be exercises. It really made me reflect on just how much trust is put in doctors and how much responsibility they have. It also made me consider the social implications of health and how much counselling doctors do. The exercise was supposed to make us approach patients holistically and it really did! I felt emotionally drained after those sessions and the pressure of ten other students watching your consultation was quite nerve wracking.

Least valuable experience

This question is really hard! There have been many times where I was sat in a three hour histology session and thought 'Why am I here?!'. However, there is a huge difference between being bored and believing something isn't very valuable. I know histology is important, I just wish it didn't have to take so long. The least valuable experiences I've had are probably some of the practical lab sessions. There were a few sessions that were quite complex, therefore everyone was getting the procedure wrong and we got rubbish results. I completely understood the reasoning behind them, but they ended up being a huge waste of time!

The future

I love thinking about the future and making lots of plans, which is probably why I find it hard to live for the day. In ten-years' time, I hope to be married and possibly a mum. I would like to have travelled the world and experienced different cultures. I hope to still be passionate about medicine and love my job. I hope to be a registrar in a specialty that I enjoy. I'm always changing my mind about the specialty I want to pursue, but I've been toying with the possibility of Obstetrics and Gynaecology or Endocrinology. I love Bioethics, so hopefully I'll be able to do some ethical research too.

I sometimes doubt whether medicine is a career that can accommodate all my hopes and aspirations. My friends all said I was stupid to go into such a competitive career when I want to have a big family, as taking time out will leave me trailing behind. Who cares! I would rather have a family than become the best consultant in the world, because I want to have a balanced life. I think you can achieve anything if you want it enough. Plus, I met an amazing female surgeon with four children and she reinforced my beliefs. She said having everything is hard, but nothing worth doing is ever easy. Wise words!

Ten things I wish I had known before starting medical school

The only thing I wanted to know before starting medical school was whether I was clever enough to make it through. I had got as far as passing my A levels and getting a place and I really wanted assurance that I would be ok. I was happy not knowing what the other aspects of medical school would be like, as it was exciting! I didn't want any preconceived opinions, because I wanted to experience everything for myself. This sounds very idealistic, but it was really to stop me being anxious. The less I knew, the less I could worry about it.

Practical Guidance Tips

- I decided to share my personal experiences of medical school, because I want to assure prospective medical students that the hard work does pay off. Coming to medical school is the best decision I've made and I hope reading this book encourages you to make the right choice.

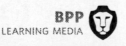